Other books of interest

Child Psychiatry
R. Goodman and S. Scott
0–632–03885–3

Clinical Paediatric Dietetics
Edited by V. Shaw and M. Lawson
0–632–03683–4

Child Health Care Nursing
Concepts, Theory and Practice
Edited by B. Carter and A. Dearmun
0–632–03689–3

The Burford NDU Model
Caring in Practice
Edited by C. Johns
0–632–03886–1

Models, Theories and Concepts
Advanced Nursing Series
Edited by J.P. Smith
0–632–03867–5

Nursing Adolescents:
Research and Psychological Perspectives
J. Taylor and D. Müller
0–632–03625–7

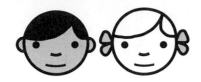

Children's Nursing in Practice
The Nottingham Model

Fiona Smith

RGN/RSCN Diploma in Professional Nursing Studies BA (Hons)/Senior Sister, Children's Accident and Emergency/The University Hospital, Queen's Medical Centre, Nottingham

with

Nottingham Children's Nurses

**Blackwell
Science**

© 1995 by
Blackwell Science Ltd
Editorial Offices:
Osney Mead, Oxford OX2 0EL
25 John Street, London WC1N 2BL
23 Ainslie Place, Edinburgh EH3 6AJ
238 Main Street, Cambridge
    Massachusetts 02142, USA
54 University Street, Carlton
    Victoria 3053, Australia

Other Editorial Offices:
Arnette Blackwell SA
1, rue de Lille, 75007 Paris
France

Blackwell Wissenschafts-Verlag GmbH
Kurfürstendamm 57
10707 Berlin, Germany

Blackwell MZV
Feldgasse 13, A-1238 Wien
Austria

First published 1995

Set by DP Photosetting, Aylesbury, Bucks
Printed and bound in Great Britain by
    the University Press, Cambridge

DISTRIBUTORS

Marston Book Services Ltd
PO Box 87
Oxford OX2 0DT
(*Orders:* Tel: 01865 791155
         Fax: 01865 791927
         Telex: 837515)

North America
Blackwell Science, Inc.
238 Main Street
Cambridge, MA 02142
(*Orders:* Tel: 800 215-1000
              617 876-7000
         Fax: 617 492-5263)

Australia
Blackwell Science Pty Ltd
54 University Street
Carlton, Victoria 3053
(*Orders:* Tel: 03 347-5552)

A catalogue record for this title
is available from the British Library

ISBN 0–632–03909–4

Library of Congress
Cataloging-in-Publication Data

Smith, Fiona.
    Children's nursing in practice: the
Nottingham model/Fiona Smith with
Nottingham children's nurses.
        p. cm.
    Includes bibliographical references and
index.
    ISBN 0–632–03909–4
    1. Pediatric nursing. 2. Family nursing.
3. Nursing models. I. Title.
    [DNLM: 1. Pediatric Nursing. 2. Patient
Care Planning. 3. Models, Nursing.
WY 159 S647c 1995]
RJ245.S585   1995
610.73'62—dc20
DNLM/DLC
for Library of Congress   94-23687
                                      CIP

On behalf of the Children's Unit in Nottingham, with due respect to the contribution of those mentioned in the acknowledgements, written, compiled and edited by Fiona Smith:

For all those children and their families, past and present, as well as in the future, who have or will be cared for within the Children's Unit in Nottingham, and for whom the model encapsulates the optimum approach to care; and for all paediatric nurses everywhere who seek to enhance practice so as to provide the ideal and optimum level of service for children and families in their care.

'This is not the end. It is not even the beginning of the end. But it is perhaps the end of the beginning.'

Winston Churchill

Contents

Preface

Over recent years, there has been an increasing interest in nursing theories and models, as well as in their application to practice. It has become very popular to develop a model that exemplifies one's practice. Many nurses, however, still find it difficult to relate models to their everyday work [1–2]. This is partly due to the vast amount of theoretical work which is more often than not written in a style which is incomprehensible and full of jargon. Therefore, when developing and writing a model upon which practice is to be based, it is imperative that it is written using simple terminology, in a style that is easily understandable and in a way that allows practitioners to relate the components to their clinical practice. The model must also be seen to be relevant to the area of clinical practice. In other words the model must be seen to be user-friendly.

Riehl and Roy [3] define a model of nursing as:

> '. . . a systematically constructed, scientifically based, and logically related set of concepts which identify the essential components of nursing practice, together with the theoretical basis of the concepts and [the] values required for their use by the practitioner.'

However, in much simpler terms a model can be described as a conceptual framework which represents a way of thinking about what nursing is, and is essentially concerned with what nurses do and how they do it. In many respects each individual nurse has his/her own model of working, which is determined by personal beliefs, values, goals and assumptions. However, in order to reach consistency in the approach to care, thereby preventing confusion and multiplicity, a collective way of thinking upon which all base their clinical practice needs to be clearly identified and agreed.

Many, however, feel that models are not required within nursing and that their use does not necessarily influence practice [4–6]. Others, such as Faucett *et al.* [7], take a different stance and argue that the use of a model not only influences practice but also quite clearly demonstrates vast improvements, such as a comprehensiveness in the approach to assessment and increased patient participation. Nevertheless, confusion continues to exist over the difference between a model of nursing and the process of nursing. The following definition identifies not only the difference but also the interdependence:

> 'A model tells us what the nursing care should be like; the nursing process describes how it should be organized.' [2]

However, it should be noted that ultimately it is the model that acts as guidance for using the process of nursing.

This book aims to demonstrate the importance of a model upon which practice is based within one children's unit. It is hoped that its use will lead to a harmonized approach to care, whether the child is nursed at home or in hospital, by a named nurse, primary nurse, specialist or community nurse. The model portrayed here essentially focuses upon two important concepts – that of care being centred on the child and family, and that of negotiated care.

The book has been written to guide practitioners working in the Nottingham Children's Unit. The emphasis is therefore towards the practical application of the model. However, as the purpose of the book is to encourage practitioners to provide the 'best' care possible for sick children and their families it is hoped that it will inspire others to also re-think and review their practice.

References

1. Clarke, D. (1986) Planning for the patient. *Senior Nurse*, **4**(5), 23–4.
2. Walsh, M. (1991) *Models in Clinical Nursing: The Way Forward*. Baillière Tindall, London.
3. Riehl, J.P. & Roy, C. (1980) *Conceptual Models for Nursing Practice*. Appleton-Century-Crofts, Norwalk.
4. Hardy, L.K. (1986) Identifying the place of theoretical frameworks in an evolving discipline. *Journal of Advanced Nursing*, **11**, 103–7.
5. Luker, K. (1988) Do Models Work? *Nursing Times*, **84** (5), 27–9.
6. Krisjanson, L.J. & Tamblyn, R. (1987) A model to guide the development and application of multiple nursing theories. *Journal of Advanced Nursing*, **12**, 523–9.
7. Faucett, J., Ellis, V., Underwood, P., Naqvi, A. & Wilson, D. (1980) The effects of Orem's self-care model in a nursing home setting. *Journal of Advanced Nursing*, **15**, 659–66.

Acknowledgements

Although it is impossible to name each individual person, an expression of thanks must be made to all those who have commented and offered their suggestions so freely, as well as to those involved in the various working groups from whom the book has benefited. Nevertheless, Sharon Stower and Angie Walker deserve to receive a mention for their input during preliminary discussions; and Marion Braley, Helen Swain and Kathleen Fleming for their contribution during the production of this book, particularly in relation to the case studies used to illustrate the model in practice. A special mention, however, must also go to Elizabeth Fradd, for the patience, encouragement and insight she offered throughout; and to Anne Marie Rafferty for her comments and advice during the final stages of production.

On a personal basis, I would like to thank all the staff in the Children's Accident and Emergency Department. I feel privileged to be part of such a caring team, for without their help and support over the last two years this book would never have been completed. Special thanks should also be made to my family, close personal friends and the publishers, for without their encouragement, support and understanding I may never have succeeded in completing the final manuscript.

Fiona Smith

Introduction

> 'Caring about or for someone is perhaps the greatest thing of all . . . but what really matters the most is actually showing them that you care not only by what you do but how you do it.'
>
> F. Smith

Over the past ten years the Children's Unit in Nottingham has striven to adapt, create and develop innovative practice to meet the needs of children and their families. This includes the development of a framework within which parents, families and professionals work together to provide the optimum care for each individual child or young person. As a result, the need to maintain an integrated approach to our care and nursing records became increasingly apparent.

In order to do so, it was necessary to identify a model or system of care that would cater for the needs of all our client groups, whether nursed in hospital, at home or in clinic (Children's Out-patients), by a primary, specialist or community nurse. The outcome of research into a variety of nursing models highlighted the fact that our needs were not met exclusively by any one of the recognized models. The decision was therefore made to pursue the development of our own model of caring, the end result of which can be seen to encompass to some extent certain elements from existing models, such as those of Roper, Logan and Tierney [1], Orem [2] and Roy [3].

It should be noted that whilst the case studies have drawn upon the author's and others' past experience, they are not related to specific cases in real life.

Terminology

The term 'child' is used to denote infants, children and young people. Unless otherwise stated the term 'parent' refers to the child's normal carer(s), as well as the family and significant others. The term 'family' extends to incorporate all those who matter the most to an individual child. The terms 'primary', 'named' and 'key' nurse are used synonymously throughout the text (refer to the Glossary for clarification of this nurse's role).

References

1. Roper, N., Logan, W. & Tierney, A. (1990) *The Elements of Nursing*, 3rd ed. Churchill Livingstone, Edinburgh.
2. Orem, D.E. (1980) *Nursing Concepts of Practice*, 2nd ed. McGraw Hill, New York.
3. Roy, C. (1976) *Introduction to Nursing: An Adaptation Model.* Prentice Hall, New Jersey.

Part 1
Developing the Model

Chapter 1
Striving for Excellence

Introduction

The purpose of this chapter is to highlight factors that have either promoted, inhibited or contributed towards the development of the Nottingham model of care. Factors affecting the achievement of significant change in nursing practice are also outlined. It should, however, be noted that the model, which centres around two important concepts – that of a child and family focused approach to care and negotiated care – is presented in chapter 2.

The Children's Unit in Nottingham upholds the philosophy and principles encompassed within publications such as *The Welfare of Children and Young People in Hospital* [1] and *Children First* [2]. The high profile the Unit has at both a national and international level has been achieved as a result of publications in the nursing press depicting developments, the close links with national bodies such as the Royal College of Nursing Society of Paediatric Nursing, international lecture tours and an annual paediatric conference in Nottingham.

Looking back

'The process of change is not just a sequence. It is a process fuelled by a variety of interpretations, each of which provides the spur to action, creates the vision and sustains the energies of those participants caught up in the process of change.' [3]

The majority of initiatives that have occurred within the unit over the last ten years, rather than being part of an overall strategic plan, have evolved gradually in response to the needs of children and families. Nurses have re-evaluated and altered their practice accordingly so as to develop, enhance and promote those issues central to the key concepts incorporated within a child and family focused approach to care. It is therefore important to stress that one should not overlook nor underestimate the amount of energy or the length of time it takes to achieve significant changes within nursing practice, particularly when resources are limited and initiatives necessitate a considerable change in attitudes, as well as the values and beliefs of those involved.

Claxton [4] describes beliefs as fixed assumptions that individuals have about the way things are in reality or the way they feel they ought to be ideally. An individual's personal commitment to his/her beliefs can lead to considerable resistance when these are threatened or challenged by innovation. Hassard and Sharifi [5] and others [6–8] indicate that any change that involves altering people's beliefs and assumptions is not only very time-consuming and expensive, but also extremely difficult to achieve.

Leading writers [5–11] on organizational change highlight the importance of certain factors upon the achievement of change that is aimed at altering culture. One of the most significant and crucial factors is leadership.

Leadership

There are almost as many definitions of leadership as there are persons who have attempted to define the concept [12]. Leadership is seen as:

> '... the ability to identify a goal, come up with a strategy for achieving that goal and inspire your team to join you in putting that strategy into action.' [13]

Essentially, therefore, it is leaders who point the way forward and inspire others to follow, whilst setting the underlying culture of any organization. Indeed, Hunt [14] states that:

> 'Leadership should be about speed, commitment, movement and releasing energy in an innovative, risk-taking environment.'

Although one would not wish to detract from the considerable influence of staff at all levels of the unit, as well as parents, families and the children themselves, much of the impetus for change can be attributed and tracked back to 1983 when Elizabeth Fradd was appointed as Divisional Nurse Manager. Essentially, it is under her guidance and as a result of her support and willingness to take risks that staff have been encouraged to be creative and to develop and enhance their practice. Hunt [14] and others [15–18] indicate that those in influential positions must not only encourage imaginative thinking and support new ideas, but also actively encourage a questioning attitude amongst staff. The latter, however, can be extremely threatening and requires a considerable degree of self-assurance and confidence, particularly when one's new beliefs and values eventually come to be challenged by enthusiastic staff advocating more radical and extensive change than originally imagined.

There are numerous constraints inhibiting the creation of an environment that promotes excellence, not least the ever increasing economic pressures related to securing sufficient funding to enable developments to take place. The failure by many to fully appreciate the value of a child and family focused approach to care has been one of the major difficulties encountered within this particular unit. Achieving significant change within nursing practice is therefore a journey fraught with many hurdles and difficulties. Machiavelli [19] states:

'It should be borne in mind that there is nothing more difficult to handle, more doubtful of success, and more dangerous to carry through than initiating changes in a state's constitution. The innovator makes enemies of all those who prospered under the old order, and only lukewarm support is forthcoming from those who would prosper under the new.'

Gaining commitment and developing a shared vision

The quote from Machiavelli above [19] highlights the fact that in order to achieve significant change within nursing practice it is imperative that one gains commitment from all those involved. It also entails creating the conditions and a vision that will sustain that commitment. Developing a shared commitment to change is one of the crucial factors underpinning the success of Nursing Development Units such as Tameside and Burford [17, 20–22].

The adoption of the key elements contained within the Children's Charter devised by the National Association for the Welfare of Children in Hospital (NAWCH) (now known as Action For Sick Children) [23] and the development of a philosophy of nursing assisted in creating a vision about the nature of the service which the Unit aimed to achieve. The key components include creating an environment that is as homelike as possible and encouraging parental/family involvement in the delivery of care.

In the early days, the process of change within the Unit could be described as a 'top-down' approach, initiatives stemming from and under the direct control of senior personnel. Those within clinical areas had little say or opportunity to express their views. Clinical staff were often not involved or consulted and therefore they were unable to influence the future direction of the Unit or the developments themselves. 'Top-down' approaches, however, only lead to resistance and non-compliance, resulting in a failure to achieve the desired alteration in the underlying beliefs and assumptions of those involved. Wright [24] and others [21, 25–26] argue that in order to achieve effective and significant change in nursing practice, all members of staff must be actively involved in planning and shaping developments.

However, it should be noted that the staff must possess the necessary skills, knowledge and confidence in order to participate fully within the change process. Continuing education and development opportunities are therefore vital in order to facilitate increased involvement. In this respect, the alteration in approach has occurred as staff have attained the confidence and ability to innovate and actively participate in shaping the developments within the Unit.

Gradually the hierarchical approach has therefore altered, so that today there is evidence of greater democracy and involvement. Staff at all levels have assumed a greater role in shaping not only developments but also the future direction of the Unit as a whole. Greater 'ownership' has been achieved, as wards and departments have devised their own philosophy in keeping with the overall philosophy of the Unit. Each year they not only set their aims and objectives for the coming year, but also evaluate the level of progress and achievement within their own area. The staff themselves are also actively involved in devising audit tools, setting standards of care and monitoring the quality of the service provided within their individual areas.

Over recent years, working groups aimed at developing practice within specific areas have evolved as a means of bringing about effective change. Staff at all levels act as representatives for their individual area, formulating, promoting, facilitating and disseminating ideas regarding developments and potential improvements in the service. These groups now act as the steering force behind the majority of the developments occurring within the Unit today.

Staff development

> ' "Staff development" refers to all those activities supported and enabled by the organization which contribute to professional and personal development.' [27]

The standard and quality of patient care are seen to be inextricably linked to the education of staff [28]. Therefore, the recognition of the need for and emphasis placed upon the provision of development opportunities for all levels of staff is one of the critical factors that underpins the significant changes that have been made within the Unit over the last ten years. Indeed, Wright [29] states that, 'Nursing cannot be developed unless nurses are given the opportunity to develop.' However, as Short [30] indicates, '... helping staff to develop ... is not just about sending them on courses ...', it is also about creating a culture and environment in which staff are supported, motivated and encouraged to learn and develop; and in which they are therefore not afraid to take risks and make mistakes.

The introduction of Individual Performance Review to identify an individual's needs, as well as the establishment of development programmes for all levels of staff within the Unit, has therefore been a means of improving patient care, changing attitudes and beliefs, and challenging accepted practice. Staff are encouraged to access formal and informal courses, with specified personnel responsible for continuing education and professional development, assisting nurses to develop, enhance and question their practice, and thereby identify areas for improvement. Continuing education and regular updates also act as a means by which to motivate staff and encourage the acceptance of change. The introduction of personal professional profiles has added to this by reinforcing the fact that individual nurses are accountable and responsible for developing and maintaining the level of their knowledge and skills.

Recruitment and retention

> 'There is strong evidence that both the numbers of nurses present and the proportion of them who are fully trained have an influence on the quality of care which can be delivered to patients.' [31]

Studies such as that by Carr-Hill *et al.* [32] highlight that the higher the grade of the nurse the better the quality of care provided. Higher standards of care and higher levels of patient satisfaction are evident in areas where patient care is delivered by trained nurses under a primary nursing system, with unqualified staff being utilized to support the qualified, rather than actually being involved directly in the delivery of patient care [20–21, 33–35]. The quality of care can therefore be enhanced not only by providing continuing education and development opportunities for all levels of staff but also by employing a higher proportion of qualified staff so as to facilitate developments such as primary nursing. However, Harper [36] states that, 'The quality of a service can only be as high as the competence level of the person providing that service.' Therefore it also equates that nurses within any area must possess the appropriate skills and expertise. In respect of paediatrics, a number of reports [1–2, 37–38] stress that children who are sick require specialist nurses with different skills and knowledge compared to those working in other fields of practice. The Audit Commission in particular highlights this by stating that:

'Nursing children differs from nursing adults in two important respects:

- the skills required to nurse the child, such as in observation techniques and psychological support, are different;
- involving parents in care requires special skills in teaching and support.' [2]

In support of these principles the Department of Health has set a standard that there should be:

'. . . *at least two* Registered Sick Children's Nurses (RSCN) (or nurses who have completed the child branch of Project 2000) on duty *24 hours a day* in all hospital children's departments and wards . . . and an RSCN available 24 hours a day to advise on the nursing of children in other departments.' [1]

Over the last 10 years, a concerted effort has been made to not only increase the proportion of RSCNs within the Children's Unit in Nottingham, but also to attract and retain high calibre individuals with the appropriate skills and ability to innovate. Numerous studies [39–44] highlight the importance of recruiting 'the right person for the job', particularly at sister level. More recently, the Allitt Inquiry [45] identified the importance of leadership and the crucial impact that the ward sister has upon standards within clinical areas. It is this individual who has the most influence on the organization and quality of patient care at ward level. Establishing two individuals at sister level (GI and GII roles in accordance with the Clinical Grading Criteria) in each clinical area, the creation of specialist posts, as well as continuing education and development opportunities, have undoubtedly influenced the quality of the service and the developments that have occurred, and have assisted in the retention of highly specialized and well-educated nurses capable of leading and shaping the future direction of the Unit.

Leenders [46] describes the 'magnet factor' – centres of excellence, which experience no difficulty in attracting and retaining staff. The philosophy within such areas is towards caring not only for the patients and relatives but also the staff. This can sometimes be difficult to achieve, which may have a considerable impact upon the quality of patient care, as well as the retention of high calibre individuals. It is therefore imperative that the environment and 'culture' reflect that depicted in the model. Staff should be involved in decision-making, feel valued, supported and given the opportunity to develop their knowledge and skills.

The widespread recognition of the Children's Unit in Nottingham has meant that the recruitment of appropriately qualified staff has become less problematic. However, there are still difficulties experienced in achieving the Department of Health's standard, despite the fact that today 98% of all trained staff hold either the RSCN qualification or have completed the Child Branch of Project 2000. The proportion of qualified to unqualified staff has altered, thereby reflecting the degree of commitment and importance attached towards ensuring that children and their families have access to and receive specialist care from appropriately qualified staff, as well as the necessary support and teaching which are considered to be vital in order to promote their full participation within the caring process.

The development of the model

'A model is not an academic exercise but must be rooted in and determined by nursing practice.' [24]

The Nottingham model reflects the philosophy of the Unit and is an attempt to rationalize the many developments that have occurred. It highlights the beliefs, values and goals that underpin nursing practice as it is today, and provides a theoretical basis for practitioners. It is also an attempt to reduce the theory–practice gap which had become increasingly evident over recent years.

Although many authors [47–50] have previously highlighted a divergence between those theories taught in the classroom and those underpinning practice, the developments occurring within this particular Unit further compounded and exacerbated a situation that to some extent already existed. The result was conflict between those theories taught by nurse educationalists regarding how nursing ought to be practised and the reality of practice in clinical areas. This situation was compounded by the fact that whilst groups of nurses within the Unit had developed a philosophy of nursing care, as well as the nursing records contained within this book, there had been until recently a failure to establish a theoretical and conceptual framework to underpin practice. Prior to the establishment of the latter, many practitioners viewed the formal theoretical knowledge taught in the school of nursing as irrelevant and not applicable to the practice area as it did not relate to the nursing records and the way nursing was practised in reality. The absence of an underlying theoretical framework also meant that educationalists tended to attach less value and significance to the practical knowledge of practising nurses concerning the way in which they conducted their everyday work.

In part, the difficulties concerning the gap between theory and practice have tended to arise from the fact that the majority of current nursing theory tends to be too abstract and context-free, and is written using obscure and incomprehensible terminology. Speedy [51] and others [52–54], indicate that the main problem stems from the fact that the majority of nursing theory is written and developed by academics who fail to appreciate the reality of nursing practice within clinical areas. Miller [55] indicates that:

> '. . . theory . . . grounded in and closely applied to nursing practice has far better potential for improving the effectiveness and the knowledge base of nursing practice and for reducing gaps between theory, practice and research than theories generated outside practice and then applied to practice.'

It would therefore seem that in order for theory to be more relevant to practitioners, as well as usable within practice areas, the development of nursing knowledge and theory must be derived from actual practice and practitioner-led.

In view of the above, the author with assistance from those named in the acknowledgements, has striven to develop a theoretical and conceptual framework so as to guide and enhance the delivery of care within the Children's Unit in Nottingham. The development of the model has resulted from reflection upon practice and a vision of an ideal. It has been led by practitioners and reflects the values, beliefs and goals underpinning a child and family focused approach to care. The importance of involving nurse educationalists within the process and the value of their input cannot be overlooked. Their involvement has had a considerable effect, particularly upon the reduction of the previously existing gap between theory and practice. Today, the nursing records utilized to apply the model in practice form the basis of much of the theoretical input within the college of nursing, and as such have been found to be an extremely useful tool whereby theory and practice can be interlinked.

Nevertheless, it should be stressed that in order to develop nursing theory and conceptual models, practitioners must be allowed time to 'think', as well as to reflect upon and to question their practice. The importance of enabling this process to occur must be acknowledged by those within senior positions, thereby allowing practitioners the time to develop theory which is derived from practice. However, in many units there is a lack of commitment from senior personnel, with enthusiastic and keen practitioners undertaking those activities related to the development of nursing theory and knowledge within their own personal time. It would seem therefore that until such activities are given equal weighting to those related to what Gray and Forsstrom [54] term 'real' nursing, many practitioners exhausted from the latter may be neither willing nor able to devote the enormous amount of time, commitment and energy that is required.

Evaluating achievement

'Excellent firms don't believe in excellence – only in constant improvement and constant change.' [56]

Although there have undoubtedly been many advances within the Children's Unit in Nottingham over the last ten years, developments continue to evolve as nurses re-evaluate and reflect upon their practice and the environment within which care is delivered. There are and always will be improvements which can be made.

In order to maintain and achieve a high standard of service that is reflective of the needs of children and their families, it is becoming increasingly important to establish and seek their views and perceptions, as well as to involve them within forums concerning developments and the future direction of the Unit. Two studies [57–58] which sought to gain an insight into parents' perceptions of the information and preparation they received, as well as their involvement in care delivery, highlighted that they felt increasingly involved and included in decision-making concerning their sick or injured child. Several of the comments made by parents stressed the value of a child and family focused approach to care and the importance of being involved in care delivery:

'... our toddler has been resident with my husband, myself and baby ... and has been cared for as much as if she was a patient herself ... we as a family think ... the 'family approach' is very welcoming ...' [58]

'... I was able to look after my child as though we were at home ... I found it very reassuring being encouraged to assist with his care ... my opinions were listened to and respected.' [58]

'Staff explained I could do as much as possible to care for my child if I wished ... the extent of which was at my discretion ...' [58]

'We were asked by the nurse what level of involvement we wanted to participate in with our child ... [this was] very useful and helpful ... both my child and myself benefited from being able to help with the care.' [58]

The above studies also indicated that in the Nottingham Unit participation in care was not always negotiated, with the result that some parents felt abandoned and unsupported in delivering care. Although the latter study [58] suggested that there had been improvements, particularly in relation to the negotiation of parents' involvement during the admission procedure,

Chandler [63] and others [64–66] also stress the importance of:

- A collegial organizational structure
- An empowering culture
- Support from senior personnel
- Good communication

- Research and professional development
- Access to information
- Recognizing and appreciating each individual's contribution.

The impact of many of the above factors upon the development of the Nottingham model has already been highlighted earlier in this chapter. The model itself emphasizes the importance of recognizing and appreciating the value of parents' knowledge concerning their child. It is considered essential that nurses build a relationship with parents that is characterized by mutual trust and respect, and within which each participant's abilities are recognized and their contribution equally valued. However, in order for that to occur and for nurses to be willing to relinquish control, they themselves must feel valued and treated with mutual respect by their superiors, as well as by members of the multi-disciplinary team. Nurses must also feel empowered in order that they are able to empower others within the caring process [67]. Empowerment is a process and outcome that is seen to arise from appreciating and valuing others.

Many large organizations, however, do not value their staff quite as much as they profess, and instead, '. . . continue merely to pay lip service to the much voiced claim that "staff are our most important resource".' [68] Often staff are not respected, with the result that they are not trusted to exercise their own judgement outside a set of highly restrictive parameters. The focus tends to be upon restricting and controlling their endeavours rather than enabling and supporting them. In many instances this may be due to a fear of losing control over the staff themselves, budgets, project work or standards. Empowerment, however, is not about losing control, but about giving it away, in order to enhance the quality of the service, whilst utilizing the skills and knowledge of one's staff to the full. Empowerment therefore involves devolving not just tasks but also decision-making and full responsibility too.

In many instances, however, there is a failure to use or harness the knowledge and understanding that even quite junior members of staff have about the needs of children, parents and families. Many senior personnel lack the confidence to take risks, focusing instead upon setting practice in rules. Whilst it is appreciated that there will always be the need for some basic and simple rules, particularly in relation to the boundaries of discretion, true empowerment is said to only operate when there are as few rules as possible. Therefore, in order to create the climate and culture that is necessary to establish and sustain the caring approach incorporated within the model, senior personnel must focus upon achieving the right balance of loose versus tight management structures and controls.

The structure must be characterized by trust and promote autonomy, with senior personnel providing support without controlling. It must include mechanisms that facilitate and promote the participation of all staff

several of the comments made suggest that some parents felt exc
from participating within certain aspects of care.

Promoting the concept of negotiated care

It is recognized that the negotiation of the level of parents' involvem
core component of partnership approaches to care. The centra
involved relate to the balance of 'power' and 'control' between hea
professionals and parents. Indeed, the perceived power imbalanc
stems from different knowledge bases has led many to question w
truly equal partnership can ever be fully established. However, the
of the opinion that equal partnerships can be established betwe
care professionals and parents, but this is dependent upon the
held by health care professionals concerning the value they att
ferent types of knowledge. A truly equal partnership is attaina
professionals view knowledge held by parents/carers regarding
to be of equal value to that held by themselves.

However, nurses do not always recognize and appreciate t
parents' knowledge regarding their child. Research sugges
recognition of parents' knowledge and capabilities varies acco
grade of nurse and the level of their experience [59–60].
experienced and the more senior the nurse the more likely
value parents' knowledge and to negotiate the level of partic
them. Therefore, it would seem likely that the recruitment an
highly skilled and experienced nurses has undoubtedly had
effect upon the level of parental participation and the
negotiated care within the Nottingham Unit.

In addition, the provision of continuing education opp
professional development programmes has also had a
influence. Whilst education and training opportunities a
means by which to change attitudes and beliefs, specific e
vision is vital in order to ensure that staff at all levels fully
concept and that they possess the skills to negotiate care
nition of the latter, specific workshops have been held,
examine their attitudes and beliefs towards parental parti
develop the vital skills to enable them to negotiate care
families.

Structural and cultural considerations invol
creation of a supportive climate

In order to achieve significant change in practice, the fo
be essential:

- A clear purpose and vision
- Clinical leadership
- Commitment from the
  organization

- Staff partici
- Staff develo

on an equal basis within decision-making processes. Communication must therefore be open and honest, and there must be a genuine regard for each other's well-being. The creation of such a 'culture' is, however, time-consuming and involves considerable effort in order to achieve the alteration in attitudes and the structure that is required.

As Schein [6] indicates, organizational cultures are developed and reinforced by several factors, the most significant of which is the activities to which senior personnel devote their time. It is imperative that time is allowed to meet with and listen to all levels of staff. Stewart [68] highlights the importance of 'walk the talk' – otherwise known as 'managing by walking about' – as a means to reinforce those values and beliefs considered to be important, whilst also demonstrating that staff are valued and truly cared about.

A lack of access to management support and involvement in decision-making is seen to lead to rigid and institutionalized approaches to care [69–71]. Therefore, in order to promote the concepts incorporated within this particular model, ward sisters and clinical nurses must be allowed and enabled to participate to a greater extent within the formulation of strategies concerning the future of the particular service within which they practise. In order to acknowledge the importance and value of those closest to the patient, greater collaboration and involvement of clinically based staff must be the norm rather than the exception. It is also imperative that staff at all levels are allowed, enabled and encouraged to function to their full potential, rather than restricted by role and grade demarcations. It is only within a culture that exhibits all of the above, and accords greater autonomy to individuals within the clinical setting, that the characteristics and outcomes of a model such as portrayed within the following chapters can become effectively established and accepted as the framework to guide and enhance the delivery of care.

Moving towards the ideal

Achieving the culture and structure discussed above is not impossible. However, it may be extremely difficult and take a considerable length of time to attain the ideal. Several authors [20–21, 25] highlight that the choice of management structure has a major impact upon the distribution of power, with lateral or collegiate structures exhibiting increased equality, respect and trust between different levels of staff. The Children's Unit has gone a long way towards creating the ultimate climate and structure. The establishment of primary nursing throughout this particular Unit has resulted in an alteration in the power structure within clinical areas, thereby increasing the degree of autonomy accorded to individual practitioners within the caring process.

Nevertheless, although the latter may be the case in relation to the caring process itself, senior and experienced staff within the clinical areas are often inhibited from utilizing their initiative, even in relation to those activities concerning future developments within their own clinical area.

There is a tendency for these developments to be controlled and led by those from outside the clinical areas. This results in not only a lack of 'ownership' amongst clinical staff but also a situation in which their expertise, skills and knowledge are devalued rather than promoted and enhanced. This can serve to inhibit and demotivate those high calibre individuals recruited to the Unit, with the result that they either become totally disillusioned and apathetic or else lost from the organization altogether.

Significant changes have occurred throughout the Nottingham Unit. However, it is apparent that there is a degree of incongruence between the wider 'culture' that exists and that advocated in relation to the model in chapter 2. The latter is seen to arise out of the impact of the enormous changes that have occurred within the NHS and the considerable conflict senior personnel are experiencing between professional values and aspirations and those related to the business-orientated culture emerging within the NHS. Consequently the time available for meeting with and communicating with staff in the Unit has become increasingly limited, with the result that senior nurses are less available for ward-based staff. The time available for such activities within the Nottingham Children's Unit is further compounded by the fact that the Unit is now spread over three separate geographical sites and is divided into numerous directorates.

Within the Unit, forums existed until recently, providing staff irrespective of status with the opportunity to discuss issues of concern and gain information from senior management. Whilst these venues have now been abolished due to poor attendance, the establishment of a regular newsletter has improved communication to a certain extent. Nevertheless, it is recognized that measures need to be taken to refocus upon communicating *with* staff at all levels of the Unit rather than communicating *to* them. The organizational structure and roles of personnel are currently under review in order to enhance communication and enable clinical staff to lead developments within practice areas.

The difficulties experienced in achieving the ultimate climate and structure to promote the concepts of the Nottingham model are not unique to this Unit. They are indicative of the fact that whilst values and beliefs may alter, it often takes much longer to achieve the ideal organizational structure. The achievement of the latter has undoubtedly been compounded by the impact of the NHS reforms and the lack of available resources.

Lessons learnt

'I love chaos: it is the mysterious, unknown road. It is the ever-unexpected . . . it is freedom, it is man's only hope. It is the poetic element in a dull and orderly world.' [72]

Stacey [73] challenges the belief that 'success' stems from a culture that is characterized by stability, harmony, regularity, discipline and consensus.

Instead, creativity is seen to be connected with instability, tension and conflict, and involves setting challenging aspirations and ambitions, reflecting upon experience, the toleration of ambiguity, the creation of a sense of adventure and conditions in which people can learn and act spontaneously using their own initiative. The successful are seen to 'be doing something else, usually without fully understanding what they are doing.' [73] Several factors, however, can be highlighted as having a crucial impact upon the achievement of significant change within nursing practice. These include:

- Developing and creating a 'vision', which is communicated with and shared by all those involved. Whilst a 'vision' is important, it is imperative that this does not restrict creativity, and as such should consist of broad parameters, thereby preventing the stifling of innovation. Stacey [73] indicates that a 'vision' can only be fully outlined retrospectively rather than prospectively.
- Involving, gaining commitment and developing a shared understanding amongst practitioners and members of the multi-disciplinary team, which is endorsed and supported by those in influential positions within the organization itself, and also within the local college of nursing.
- Visible leadership at not only a senior level but also within the clinical area. This includes the careful selection of the most appropriate person to lead and enhance developments. It should be noted that this may not always be a senior person, but could be a junior staff nurse with a new idea. Attention should, however, be given towards ensuring that the person has the right skills, ability and above all the motivation and commitment required to overcome the numerous obstacles that they will undoubtedly face. Ideally, project work and developments should be led by those within rather than outside the clinical areas, senior personnel enabling and supporting staff within clinical areas to do so, rather than directing and controlling such activities as has so often been the case in the past.
- Creating a 'culture' that is characterized by mutual trust and respect, and within which staff feel valued, supported and are given due recognition for their endeavours.
- Continuing education and staff development so as to achieve the desired alteration in the underlying beliefs and assumptions of those involved, as well as the means by which to facilitate staff participation within the process of change by encouraging and enabling them to develop the skills, knowledge and confidence.
- Involving users in decisions regarding the future direction of the service, which includes actively seeking their opinions, listening to and responding to their comments and suggestions.

It must be recognized that 'The seeds of the future lie in the present' [74]. Therefore one must not only be prepared to invest the time and energy in order that they may grow, but also keep one's mind constantly open to new suggestions and new ways of thinking and doing.

References

1. Department of Health (1991) *The Welfare of Children and Young People in Hospital.* HMSO, London.
2. Audit Commission (1993) *Children First.* HMSO, London.
3. Wilson, D.C. (1992) *A Strategy of Change.* Routledge, London.
4. Claxton, G. (1987) Beliefs and behaviour: Why is it so hard to change? *Nursing,* **3**, 670–3.
5. Hassard, J. & Sharifi, S. (1989) Corporate culture and strategic change. *Journal of General Management,* **15** (2), 4–19.
6. Schein, E.H. (1986) *Organisational Culture and Leadership.* Jossey-Bass, San Francisco.
7. Frost, P.J., Moore, L.F., Loius, M.R., Lundberg, C.C. & Martin, J. (1985) *Organisational Culture.* Sage, London.
8. Martin, J. & Siehl, C. (1983) Organisational Culture and Counterculture: An uneasy symbiosis. *Organizational Dynamics,* **11** (2), 52–64.
9. Ott, J.S. (1989) *The Organisational Culture Perspective.* Brooks/Cole Publishing Co., California.
10. Nadler, D.A. & Tushman, M.L. (1989) Organizational Frame Bending: Principles for Managing Reorientation. *Academy of Management Executive,* **3** (3), 194–204.
11. Brown, A. (1992) Organizational Culture: The Key to Effective Leadership and Organizational Development. *Leadership and Organization Development Journal,* **13** (2), 3–6.
12. Stogdill, R.M. (1974) *Handbook of Leadership: A Survey of Theory and Research.* Free Press, London.
13. Rafferty, A.M. (1993) *Leading Questions.* King's Fund Centre, London.
14. Hunt, J. (1992) Nursing Leadership Opportunities. *Senior Nurse,* **12** (1), 13–15.
15. Strasen, L. (1992) *The Image of Professional Nursing: Strategies for Action.* J.B. Lippincott Co., London.
16. Adair, J. (1988) *Effective Leadership.* Pan Books, London.
17. Wright, S.G. (1989) *Changing Nursing Practice.* Edward Arnold, London.
18. Vestal, K. (1988) Managing Innovation in Paediatrics. *Journal of Paediatric Nursing,* **1** (2), 124.
19. Machiavelli, N. (1961) *The Prince.* Penguin, Harmondsworth.
20. Black, M. (1993) *The Growth of Tameside Nursing Development Unit.* King's Fund Centre, London.
21. Pearson, A. (1992) *Nursing At Burford: A Story of Change.* Scutari Press, London.
22. Turner Shaw, J. & Bosanquet, N. (1993) *A Way To Develop Nurses and Nursing.* King's Fund Centre, London.
23. NAWCH (1984) *The Children's Charter.* NAWCH, London.
24. Wright, S.G. (1986) *Building and Using a Model of Nursing.* Edward Arnold, London.
25. Pearson, A. (ed.) (1988) *Primary Nursing.* Chapman & Hall, London.
26. Lancaster, J. & Lancaster, W. (1982) *The Nurse as Change Agent.* C.V. Mosby & Co., St Louis.
27. Heath, J. (1987) Who and What Influences Staff Development. *Senior Nurse,* **7** (6), 17–19.
28. Fretwell, J.E. (1985) *Freedom to Change.* Royal College of Nursing, London.

29. Wright, S.G. (1993) The historical background to the Tameside Nursing Development Unit. In: *The Growth of Tameside Nursing Development Unit*, (M. Black). King's Fund Centre, London.
30. Short, C. (1990) The Manager's Involvement. *Nursing*, **4** (8), 17–19.
31. Bagust, A. (1992) Quality or quantity. *Health Service Journal*, **102** (5314), 23–5.
32. Carr-Hill, R., Dixon, P., Gibbs, I., Griffiths, M., Higgins, M., McCaughlan, D. & Wright, K. (1992) *Skill-mix and the Effectiveness of Nursing Care.* Centre For Health Economics, University of York.
33. Pearson, A. (ed.) (1989) *Primary Nursing.* Chapman & Hall, London.
34. MacGuire, J. (1988) I'm your nurse. *Nursing Times*, **84** (30), 33–6.
35. Hegyvary, S.T. (1977) Foundations of Nursing. *Nursing Clinics of North America*, **12** (2), 185–96.
36. Harper, L. (1986) All Mixed Up. *Nursing Times*, **82** (48), 28–31.
37. Ministry of Health (1959) *The Welfare of Children in Hospital* (Platt Report). HMSO, London.
38. Report of the Committee on Child Health Services (1976) *Fit For The Future* (Court Report). HMSO, London.
39. Audit Commission (1991) *The Virtue of Patients: Making the Best Use of Ward Nursing Resources.* HMSO, London.
40. Pembrey, S. (1980) *The Ward Sister: Key to Nursing.* Royal College of Nursing, London.
41. Jeffree, C. (1988) Management, Care and the Role of the Ward Sister. *Senior Nurse*, **8** (12), 10–12.
42. Ogier, M.E. (1982) *An Ideal Sister.* Royal College of Nursing, London.
43. Fretwell, J. (1982) *Ward Teaching and Learning.* Royal College of Nursing, London.
44. Orton, H.D. (1981) *Ward Learning Climate.* Royal College of Nursing, London.
45. Report of the Independent Inquiry Relating to Deaths and Injuries on the Children's Ward at Grantham and Kesteven General Hospital During the Period February to April 1991 (1991) *The Allitt Inquiry.* HMSO, London.
46. Leenders, F. (1985) The Magnet Factor. *Nursing Times*, **81** (40), 44–5.
47. Bendall, E. (1975) *So You Passed, Nurse.* Royal College of Nursing, London.
48. Dodd, A.P. (1973) *Towards an Understanding of Nursing.* Unpublished PhD thesis, Goldsmiths College, University of London.
49. Hunt, J.M. (1974) *The Teaching and Practice of Surgical Dressings in Three Hospitals.* Royal College of Nursing, London.
50. McCaugherty, D. (1992) The gap between nursing theory and practice. *Senior Nurse*, **12** (6), 44-8.
51. Speedy, S. (1989) Theory–practice debate: setting the scene. *The Australian Journal of Advanced Nursing*, **6** (3), 12–19.
52. Conant, L. (1967) Closing the theory–practice gap. *Nursing Outlook*, **15** (11), 37–9.
53. Wald, F.S. & Leonard, R.C. (1964) Toward a development of nursing practice theory. *Nursing Research*, **13** (4), 309–13.
54. Gray, J. & Forsstrom, S. (1991) Generating theory from practice: the reflective technique. In: *Towards a Discipline of Nursing*, (eds G. Gray & R. Pratt). Churchill Livingstone, London.
55. Miller, A. (1991) Theory to practice: implementation in the clinical setting. In: *Current Issues in Nursing*, (eds M. Jolley & P. Allan). Chapman & Hall, London.

56. Peters, T. (1988) *Thriving on Chaos*. Pan Books, London.
57. Smith, F.M. (1992) *A study into parents'/carers' perceptions of the preparation and information they received, and their involvement in care delivery*. Unpublished, Children's Unit, Nottingham.
58. Smith, F.M. (1993) *A follow-up study of progress: parents'/carers' perceptions of the preparation and information they received, and their involvement in care delivery*. Unpublished, Children's Unit, Nottingham.
59. Callery, P. & Smith, L. (1991) A study of role negotiation between nurses and the parents of hospitalised children. *Journal of Advanced Nursing*, **16**, 772–81.
60. Gill, K.M. (1987) Parent Participation With a Family Health Focus: Nurses' Attitudes. *Pediatric Nursing*, **13** (2), 94–6.
61. Casey, A. (1993) Development and Use of the Partnership Model of Nursing Care. In: *Advances in Child Health Nursing* (eds E.A. Glasper & A. Tucker). Scutari Press, London.
62. Cole, A. & Vaughan, B. (1994) *Reflections Three Years On*. King's Fund Centre, London.
63. Chandler, G.E. (1991) Creating an Environment to Empower Nurses. *Nursing Management*, **22** (8), 20–23.
64. Swanwick, M. & Barlow, S. (1993/4) A Caring Definition. *Child Health*, **1** (4), 137–41.
65. Lancaster, J. (1985) Creating a Climate for Excellence. *Journal of Nursing Administration*, **15**, 16–19.
66. Gorman, S. & Clark, N. (1986) Power and Effective Nursing Practice. *Nursing Outlook*, **34** (3), 129–34.
67. Chevasse, J.M. (1992) New Dimensions of Empowerment in Nursing – and Challenges. *Journal of Advanced Nursing*, **17** (1), 1–2.
68. Stewart, A.M. (1994) *Empowering People*. Pitman Publishing, London.
69. Wright, S.G. (1993) Management as an integral part of nursing. *Journal of Nursing Management*, **1**, 129–32.
70. Martin, J.P. (1984) *Hospitals in Trouble*. Blackwell, Oxford.
71. Simpson, K. (1985) Authority and responsibility delegation predicts quality of care. *Journal of Advanced Nursing*, **10**, 345–8.
72. Shahn, B. (1966) Leadership and creativity. In: *Frontiers of Leadership* (eds M. Syrett & C. Hogg). Blackwell, London.
73. Stacey, R. (1992) *Managing Chaos*. Kogan Page, London.
74. Adair, J. (1987) *Not Bosses But Leaders*. Kogan Page, London.

Chapter 2
The Nottingham Model

Introduction

The Nottingham model centres around two main concepts: that of care being centred on the child and family and that of negotiated care. These two concepts facilitate a caring approach which is based upon the achievement of an equal partnership between professionals and the child/ parents and family. It should, however, be noted that these fundamental concepts have previously been identified by Orem [1] and that one of the bases of the model is an adaptation of Roper, Logan and Tierney's [2] Activities of Living.

Beliefs and values

A child forms part of a complex family unit and wider community, and as such can only function to his/her full potential within a stable family relationship. However, Article 13 of the United Nations Convention on the Rights of the Child (1989) states that:

> 'The child shall have the right to freedom of expression; this right shall include freedom to seek, receive and impart information and ideas of all kinds, regardless of frontiers, either orally, in writing or in print, in the form of art, or through any other media of the child's choice.' [3]

It is therefore recognized that listening to the child and involving him/her in decision-making whenever possible is extremely important in order that the child is able to retain dignity and respect. It must therefore be said that although the current philosophy of child care promotes family-centred care, the best interests of the child must be a primary consideration in all actions concerning the child's health needs [3: Article 13]. Staff working alongside parents should promote what is in the best interests of the individual child by enabling the child to express his/her views freely and ensuring that these receive consideration:

> '... in accordance with the age and maturity of the child, and that children's views must be considered and taken into account in all matters affecting them.' [3: Article 12]

Therefore, in view of the above, the imparting of information is a particularly skilled affair which requires patience and understanding from parents as well as health care professionals.

Admission to hospital and the ensuing disruption to the child's usual routine upsets the child's equilibrium, the end result of which may well be an alteration in the child's normal functioning – emotionally, physically, socially or psychologically. Research indicates that the effects of hospitalization upon a child's development can be long-term, often extending into adulthood and affecting relationships, as well as employment prospects [4–10]. It is therefore recognized that the best place for the child to be cared for is in his/her own home by his/her family whenever possible. However, when admission is required, for a child to receive optimum care, it is necessary to have a welcoming environment which promotes normal development and facilitates negotiated care throughout the child's stay in hospital and into the community when care continues at home.

Goals

Ultimately the goal is to care for the child with his/her best interests in mind [3, 11]. It is also important to maintain the integrity of the family unit, promoting care by the family and enabling them to maintain their independence and control over their lives. An essential component of this is the maintenance of the child's usual routine whenever possible during the illness, whether the child is nursed in hospital or at home (Table 2.1).

It is aimed to achieve this goal by:

● Allowing the child the freedom to express his/her views freely.
● The encouragement of parents/family to stay with their child if at all possible or to visit whenever they can.
● The provision of a 'child-friendly' atmosphere and environment which promotes dignity and independence.
● Supporting and encouraging the child and family to participate in care planning and care giving as much as they are able to or wish to.
● The establishment of a primary nursing system of organizing and delivering patient care (acknowledging the Department of Health guidance in the Patient's Charter that each patient should have access to a named nurse [12]).
● The development of an effective and appropriately skilled community nursing team, enabling children to be nursed at home whenever possible and/or discharged home at the earliest conceivable time (in recognition of the concepts underpinning the Community Care Act [13]).

Child and family focused care

Butler-Sloss in the Cleveland Inquiry notes that, 'The child is a person and not an object of concern.' [14]. Indeed, Article 3 of the United Nations

Table 2.1 The Children's Charter. Serving children in Nottingham.

- Children and their parents have a right to express things in their own way and to be involved in decision-making. We have a responsibility to preserve these rights within the operational constraints of this hospital.
- Children should have impartial access to treatment and facilities that are available within the hospital for them.
- Children have a right to considerate and respectful care, which maintains their dignity at all times.
- Children and their parents have rights of privacy and confidentiality.
- Children have the right to be treated in a safe environment.
- Communications should be clear and in plain language. An understanding by the child as well as the parent is important. Help should be given to those with communication difficulties.
- Parents are welcome to participate in the care of their children when appropriate. We have the responsibility to provide adequate support.
- Parents have the right to stay with their child during the hospital stay. Accommodation or sleeping facilities will be provided.
- Children have the right to appropriate education and play facilities during their stay in hospital.
- Children and parents are entitled to know the name and the professional status of each person providing a service for them.
- Children and their parents have a right to be consulted about care being given or involvement in teaching and research.
- Children and their families are entitled to expect communication, and liason between hospital, community health services and other caring agencies.

Convention on the Rights of the Child (1989) states that, 'In all actions concerning children ... the best interests of the child shall be a primary consideration' [3]. Article 24 concerning health and health services states that a child has the right, '... to the enjoyment of the highest attainable standard of health and to the facilities for the treatment of illness and rehabilitation of health' [3]. The 'best interests' principle is reiterated in the Children Act 1989 [11], the overriding purpose of which is to promote and safeguard the welfare of children. Documents such as *Welfare of Children and Young People in Hospital* [15] and *Children First: A Study of Hospital Services* [16] stress the fact that children require a different approach to health care provision, within an appropriate environment that facilitates child and family centred care.

The Department of Health document *Welfare of Children and Young People in Hospital* [15] states that:

'A good quality service for children ... provides for the child as a whole, for his or her complete physical and emotional well-being and not simply for the condition for which treatment is required ...'

Child health service provision and the environment within which care is delivered should therefore reflect an appreciation of the different needs of children when compared with other client groups. This includes taking into account their psychological, social, emotional and developmental needs, as well as their physical requirements, through the provision of appropriate facilities, the inclusion of their family and an approach that encourages the maintenance of each child's usual activities and routine, whether he/she receives treatment or care within a hospital setting or within the home environment.

Therefore, a good quality service is one that not only acknowledges the different needs of children via specifically written policies and standards, but also devises and adopts measures through which a child's total needs can be met irrespective of the child's treatment or care requirements. For example, the importance of play, education and peer support has been documented as a means through which the child learns, develops, expresses his/her innermost feelings and comes to terms with significant changes in his/her circumstances. Therefore, measures such as the following can be seen to go some way towards meeting a child's complete needs rather than purely focusing upon the child's physical requirements.

- The provision of bedside tuition when the child is unable to attend his/her own or hospital school enables education to continue.
- Employing nursery nurses to ensure that appropriate toys and play activities related to each child's needs, preferences and age are freely available.
- Widening doors to playrooms so that children restricted to bed can continue to play and socialize with others.
- The provision of separate recreation facilities for adolescents, encouraging the development of youth activities and peer group support.

The whole approach and central focus should be upon achieving not only a child-centred environment but a child-centred routine in respect of each child's usual sleeping and feeding patterns, recreation and learning activities, the overall aim being to facilitate the maintenance or achievement of the child's usual level of independence, activities and routine. The caring process should also reflect what is in each child's best interests. This includes recognizing and acknowledging the child's specific needs and wishes. Attention and patience must therefore be devoted to encouraging and enabling the child (according to maturity, cognitive ability and developmental level) to express his/her views and opinions quite freely, whether verbally, through play or associated activities; and involving the child in the decision-making process regarding his/her care whenever possible. This fact is reiterated in the Children Act 1989 [17] which states that, 'Children should be kept informed about what happens to them and should participate when decisions are made about their future.'

Therefore, the process of nursing itself and the conceptual framework that guides nursing practice should reflect an appreciation and recognition of the complete needs of a child, focus on the child and promote the child's best interests. The child should be involved whenever possible in the assessment and identification of his/her needs, the planning of the care, measures to meet such needs, care delivery and evaluation.

Involving a child in such activities requires a great deal of skill on the part of the practitioner and necessitates:

- The use of an appropriate pain scale related to the child's age and cognitive ability.
- The use of appropriate play and techniques to explain procedures and forthcoming events.
- The appreciation and respect of the child's parents' 'expert' knowledge concerning their child's usual behaviour and level of independence.

In order to enable a young child to participate as fully as possible within the activities involved in the caring process, the nurse must possess excellent communication and interpersonal skills, as well as a considerable amount of ingenuity.

One cannot overstate that in order for a child's needs to be met in an appropriate and optimum manner, which includes involving the child within the caring process, children should receive care from nurses who have undergone specific training to provide for their needs [15–16]. It is only with such training that a nurse will have developed both the knowledge and the skills to facilitate a child and family focused approach, thereby maintaining the integrity of the family unit as a whole [18].

The caring process and the emphasis of child health service provision should acknowledge that a child is part of a 'family', upon whom he/she is constantly dependent for physical care and emotional support. Therefore, siblings, parents/carers and the 'family' should be involved in the caring process and their need for care and support should be appreciated and acknowledged. As Jolly [19] states:

> 'The challenge of paediatric nursing today is in meeting the needs of the whole child. This means not only attending to his physical care, but also paying attention to his thoughts, his feelings, and his need for his family.'

Over recent years, the trend within nursing has been towards involving families in health care; and nowhere is this more evident than within the field of paediatrics. Indeed, terms such as 'family-centred care', 'family nursing' and 'family focused care' are frequently mentioned throughout the nursing press.

Child and family focused care is:

- Recognizing that caring for a child also includes caring for the family, in the belief that the child feels much safer and more secure when the family also feels cared about and cared for.
- Acknowledging a family's right to be involved in decision-making regarding their child's care, and a child's right to be included in discussions whenever possible.

- Respecting a family's knowledge about their child, with nurses sharing information and knowledge, so that together the nurse/child/parent and family may plan and implement the optimum care to meet the needs of the child, as well as those of the family.
- Assisting the child and family to retain control over their lives and to continue to meet their own/their child's physical, social, emotional and health care needs, by enabling and facilitating adaptation and the development of additional caring skills through teaching, advice or support, whether care is to be given within a hospital environment or at home.
- Encouraging children themselves and their family to participate in care giving as much as they wish and feel able to; and to visit or be resident with their child whenever they can, in the belief that children get better quicker when they are cared for by those they love and by whom they are loved.

It has, however, been noted that many families lack an understanding of the term child and family focused care and their role within the caring process. Explanation is therefore presented in a 'Parent and Family Information' file (a copy of which is kept by each child's bed), giving details about the Children's Unit and facilities available within and nearby the hospital, and information in relation to parental involvement in care. This includes explicitly-written guidance about what parents should expect from the nurse and what the nurse needs from them, in order that individualized and effective care is provided for the child (Table 2.2).

It can be seen that family-centred care means more than just parental involvement in care delivery, but includes caring for the whole family's needs. The key to its success lies in the empowerment of the child, parent and family through the imparting of information and knowledge in order that they are able to participate in decision-making and thereby the caring process on an equal basis.

In Nottingham, specifically designed leaflets written in easily under-standable terms with the use of diagrams as appropriate give parents information related to a variety of issues including their child's illness and treatment (see Appendix 1 for some examples). Although these are given to parents as and when appropriate, copies of all available leaflets, including others related to the prevention of illness, as well as specifically chosen texts, are available within the Family Resource Centre situated in the Children's Out-patient Department. (It should be noted that at the time of writing, this area is in the process of being commissioned.) Families are able to borrow texts from this area, as well as videos concerning treatment and procedures. This enables them to play an active role in the preparation of their child for forthcoming procedures or increase their knowledge concerning any aspect of their child's needs.

However, each individual parent/family's ability to cope with their child's period of illness and the change in their circumstances varies according to their support network and the coping methods and strategies available to them. As such, a multi-disciplinary approach is utilized to meet

Table 2.2 An extract from the Parent and Family Information File.

You can expect your primary nurse to:

● Get to know you, your child and family.
● Plan with you the nursing care to meet your child's needs.
● Explain the plans to the associate nurse who will care for your child when your primary nurse is off-duty.
● Tell you what to expect before tests or treatments.
● Teach you about health care related to your child's illness.
● Arrange follow-up and liaise with your health visitor, district nurse and social worker.

We need you to:

● Tell your nurse what you want.
● Keep your nurse informed about how you feel.
● Tell your nurse if you have an idea or a preference about your child's nursing care.

Your nurse will:

● Encourage you to participate in caring for your child as much as you wish and feel able to.
● Discuss the level of your involvement with you.
● Ask you to participate in planning your child's care and to sign the plan of care to demonstrate that this has been discussed with you.

We need you to:

● Tell us if there is something that you would like to undertake or if there is something that you would prefer not to do.

Please do not feel that you must carry out your child's care at all times or feel pressurized in any way.

Please help us to help you by telling your nurse how you feel and letting him/her know when you would like assistance or a 'break'.

their needs, the child and family's named nurse acting as the main pivot, identifying their unique needs and refering to and involving other professionals in the child and family's care where appropriate. (The importance of this nurse is explored later in this chapter.)

In Nottingham, family care assistants arrange accommodation and assist parents and families during their child's stay in hospital. In addition, professional advice, counselling and support is available from paediatric liaison health visitors; and social workers assist with issues such as financial or transportation difficulties, as well as child care arrangements for other siblings or measures to ensure the continuation of the latter's education.

Information and preparation for hospital admission

Admission to hospital is a time of anxiety and fear of the unknown for the family as well as for the child. However, anxieties and fears can be substantially reduced by preparation, as well as the provision of information. It has been well documented that receiving adequate information concerning treatment and the experience of hospitalization aids recovery by reducing anxiety and stress amongst patients [20–23]. Numerous studies indicate that children who receive preparation prior to admission are less anxious, more co-operative, better able to adapt to their new surroundings, more likely to make a speedier recovery and are also less likely to display behavioural and emotional disturbance following discharge [24–31]. Therefore, it is extremely valuable and worthwhile to prepare children for admission to hospital and for procedures they will encounter.

The importance of providing adequate preparation and information for parents and carers has also been highlighted [32–34]. It is they who provide security, as well as continuity, for the child in an otherwise strange and unfamiliar environment. However, if they themselves are anxious they may be unable to provide this sense of security for their child. As Vernon [34] states:

> 'Anxious parents are less capable of providing security for children in a time of stress ... and that anxiety may interfere with effective psychological preparation for hospital and surgery.'

Therefore, preparing the parent as well as the child is extremely important, especially as parental anxieties can not only be mirrored in the child but also exacerbate fear and feelings of insecurity [25–26]. Yet Harris [35] and others [36–37] indicate that many parents often feel unprepared for the planned admission of their child to hospital or for any procedures they will experience. As a result they feel unable to prepare their child and to answer their child's questions or alleviate his/her fears.

In 1976 the Court Report [38], recognizing the importance of preparing young children for admission to hospital, expressed concern over the fact that, '... much more could be done in practice to reduce the risk of hospital admission being psychologically highly stressful for children.' The Report recommended an increase in the number of pre-admission programmes offered to children and their families. However, although there has been a gradual increase in the number of children's units offering these programmes [25, 36, 39–40], there are many others that continue to pay mere lip service to the need for preparation and do so solely by the provision of booklets for parents. Although, provision of the latter is undoubtedly a useful source of information, the importance of a preadmission programme that incorporates a visit to ward areas along with additional information should not be underestimated.

Pre-admission programmes

Pre-admission programmes are concerned with stress innoculation [41]. Meng and Zastowny [24] indicate that stress innoculation involves:

- education regarding the nature of stress;
- introduction and development of specific coping skills; and
- practise of coping skills during exposure to stressors.

Most pre-admission programmes therefore incorporate some sort of audio-visual presentation concerning admission to hospital and procedures that will be encountered, a tour of relevant clinical areas, including in some cases the anaesthetic room, as well as an opportunity for therapeutic play. These visits enable the child and family to meet staff and familiarize themselves with the environment, and provide parents with the opportunity to seek additional information, express their anxieties and clarify their role in preparing and supporting their child.

One of the first pre-admission schemes to be developed in this country was the 'Saturday Morning Project' offered in Nottingham. This scheme is primarily aimed at those children who are due to be admitted for planned surgery. Invitations (Table 2.3) are sent to the child and parents, along with a programme (Table 2.4), the Nottingham Children's Unit preparatory booklet *At Home in Hospital*, an information leaflet concerning the relevant ward to which the child will be admitted (see Appendix 2 for some examples), and details concerning the date of admission.

Table 2.3 Invitation to the Saturday Morning Project.

Dear

You will soon be coming to stay with us in the hospital and we would like to meet you to tell you about the wards.

Please bring Mummy, Daddy and brothers and sisters to the University Hospital, Nottingham on any Saturday morning before admission. Meet in the Main Entrance, B Floor at 10 AM.

Table 2.4 outlines the itinerary for the morning, which begins with an automated tape-slide lecture showing the day of admission and the aspects of hospital life that the child will experience, following which visits are made to the ward areas to which the child will subsequently be admitted. Whilst the latter familiarizes the child with the hospital environment, the exposure to audio-visual information that depicts a child actor experiencing pre-operative procedures which the child will encounter not only decreases anxiety but also increases co-operation as the child is able to interpret these events on a 'secondhand' basis and assimilate them into his/her previous experiences [37, 42–45]. Time is also set aside during the morning for the child to play, 'dress up' and 'pretend', as well as to become familiar with items of hospital equipment such as stethoscopes. Parents are also given

Table 2.4 Programme for the Saturday Morning Project.

Nottingham Health Authority University Hospital
Children's Department Hospital Tour
Saturday mornings

Itinerary

10.00 AM	Meet in the Main Entrance, B Floor.
10.05 AM (approx.)	*Coming into Hospital* – an automated tape slide lecture showing aspects of life in hospital that affect children.
10.30 AM	Visit to ward – children may wish to see (especially) a bed, a locker, the toilets and bathroom, the TV sets and the playroom, and be introduced to the ward staff.
11.00 AM	Children's playtime – the children meet each other and play, supervized by members of the staff and volunteers.
	Meanwhile
	Parents are invited to view a video tape presentation, *The Operation*, in a nearby room. This does not show surgery being performed, but gives a child's view of the events surrounding having an operation at University Hospital.
11.20 AM	Time to ask questions or discuss particular worries of a non-medical nature.
	Parents rejoin children.
	Play-packs – issued to children expecting admission. (These items may be kept.)

---

time to ask questions of a non-medical nature and are invited to watch a video that reflects a child's view of the events surrounding having an operation, including the administration of the anaesthetic.

It can be said that it is never possible to ensure that all children are adequately prepared for admission to hospital, as not every admission is planned. However, it is possible to prepare many more for the possibility of a hospital admission, by inviting siblings to attend pre-admission programmes and by educating children at venues such as play groups, day nurseries, primary and nursery schools [46].

Nevertheless, as the majority of children are admitted as 'emergencies' due to acute episodes of illness or as a result of accidents, the need to overcome any deficit in preparation must be acknowledged by professionals during the immediate post-admission period. The provision of photographs and books depicting life in hospital in Accident and Emergency and Out-patient Departments may alleviate some of the child's and parents' anxieties prior to arrival on the ward. However, the importance of also explaining procedures and events to parents and children must not be overlooked.

The use of play materials, as well as appropriate explanations geared towards the child's level of understanding, can do much to alleviate anxiety and prepare children for procedures they will experience. Rodin [32] highlights that children who have been 'told' by their parents beforehand about a blood test not only display less anxiety but also are much more able to cope with subsequent events. Therefore, it is imperative that parents receive adequate information in order that they can prepare their child, and that they are also given the opportunity (if they wish) to be actively involved in providing explanations, as well as support, for their child throughout any procedure.

The role of play in preparing a child for procedures

Numerous publications and reports [38, 47–49], including the Department of Health document *Welfare of Children and Young People in Hospital* [15], stress the importance of providing play facilities in hospital:

'Play is essential for the normal intellectual, social and emotional development of children.' [15]

'Second to the continuing presence of the mother or another supporting figure, play can be an important factor in diminishing the harmful effects of stress in hospitalized children.' [50]

Play in hospital not only promotes normal development but also helps to reduce the detrimental psychological effects and emotional trauma associated with a period of hospitalization. Research also indicates that play reduces anxiety, facilitates communication and aids recovery as well as rehabilitation [51–52]. For example, promoting activities such as blow painting or blowing bubbles can aid breathing following surgery.

Play has often been referred to as the work of the child. It is the medium through which children learn and can express their fears and anxieties, as well as 'act out' their frustration or anger concerning unpleasant occurrences. Play also allows children to explore and gain an understanding about what is happening to them; and therefore it is a valuable tool for explaining procedures and for preparing children for experiences they will encounter. The use of games, story books, videos, pictures, diagrams and photographs, as well as toys, dolls and puppets with various attachments such as long lines, naso-gastric tubes, catheters and intravenous cannulae, all assist in this process [53–54].

It is vital for children and their parents to receive preparation and information concerning admission to hospital, as well as for any procedures they may encounter. The provision of an environment that is geared towards meeting the needs of children and that aims to maintain the child's usual routine and activities is also extremely important. Fradd [54] states that, 'Making hospital like home is vital to the success of any child's stay.' Therefore, encouraging parents to bring in their child's own clothes and other familiar belongings, including their favourite toy/comforter, as well as encouraging parents and other family members, including pets, to be resident or visit whenever they can, not only increases the child's sense of security and continuity, but also creates a degree of normality within what would otherwise be a totally strange and unfamiliar environment.

The philosophy of nursing care

The philosophy of the Children's Unit in Nottingham reflects the goals and beliefs underpinning a child and family focused approach to care (Table 2.5). This includes the provision of an environment that is appropriate for children of all ages, and open, honest communication between professionals and children and their families.

Aims

By attaining the goals incorporated within a child and family focused approach to care and the principles outlined in Nottingham's philosophy of nursing care, the traumatic effects of a period of hospitalization can either be avoided or substantially reduced. The end result is a much happier and contented child and family, which in itself leads to a speedier recovery and shorter hospital stays [7, 57–60].

The basis of the model

Core elements

Definition of health

The definition of health to which Nottingham refers is contained in the constitution of the World Health Organization, '... a state of complete physical, mental and social well-being and not merely the absence of disease or infirmity' [61]. This statement was adopted by the International Health Conference held in New York in July 1946 and was signed by representatives of 61 states.

However, 'being healthy' means different things to different people and it is therefore important for health care professionals to identify what being healthy means to each individual child and family. The Nottingham model emphasizes the importance of identifying the child's normal or usual level of independence and behaviour, as well as his/her physical and social development. The nurse therefore ascertains the child and family's perception of 'health' when gaining information in relation to the child's deviation from this norm.

This holistic approach to health takes into account the impact of factors such as culture, religion, and social/economic status, which it is recognized vary depending on an individual's beliefs and values. Figure 2.1 highlights some of the immediate and wider influences which can affect a child's health.

Table 2.5 Philosophy of nursing care in the Children's Unit.

The United Nations Convention on the Rights of the Child [3], The National Association of the Welfare of Children in Hospital (now known as Action For Sick Children) [55], together with the principles of the Children Act 1989 [56] and the standards stated in the Welfare of Children and Young People in Hospital [15] are fundamental to our philosophy and practice.

The children's nurse should:

- Acknowledge a child's unique needs and act as the child's advocate to ensure these needs are not overlooked or misunderstood.
- Respect a child's right to privacy and dignity and accept the child's right to be recognized as an individual, without discrimination in respect of disability, race, culture, language, religion or gender.
- Minimize stress and separation during visits to hospital by providing physical, emotional, social and spiritual support and should they so wish, accommodation to all families.
- Maintain a safe environment for the child and develop up-to-date care which is research-based.
- Communicate honestly and effectively with families using plain language that the child and parent can understand. Recognize the importance of assessing the child's level of understanding and create time to listen and explain. The nurse must appreciate the need to use the interpreting service where applicable.
- View parents as partners in care to the degree that they are able and wish to be involved. Encourage, support and supervise family involvement.
- Respect the wishes of parents/carers, acknowledging different cultural and religious beliefs in a non-judgemental way.
- Sensitively and imaginatively view the hospital through the eyes of the child and create an emotionally healthy environment. Provide play and education facilities to maximize the child's potential and maintain an element of normality.
- Enable children to be nursed in the most appropriate environment, including their home.
- Recognize the child as an integral part of his/her family and local community.
- Develop strong communication and liaison between team members, both in hospital and the community, to facilitate uniformity and continuity of care.
- Develop a multi-disciplinary approach to care in the community.
- Recognize and respect the unique role of each member of the health care team.
- Ensure families recognize that they have a choice as to whether or not they participate in research and teaching.

At the time of writing, the philosophy of nursing care in the Children's Unit is in the process of being updated by a multi-disciplinary group.

Fig. 2.1 Examples of the immediate and wider influences upon a child's health.

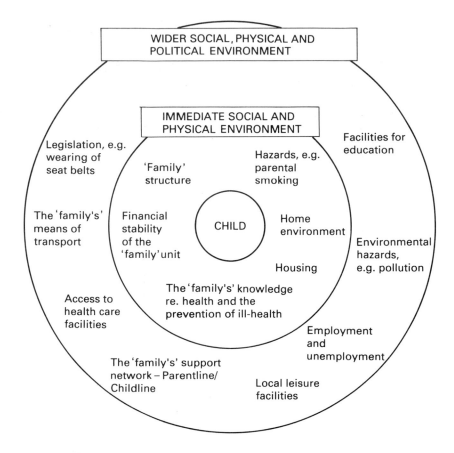

The concept of 'health' can therefore be seen to be extremely complex, consisting of different aspects which are interrelated and interdependent with each other. The different aspects or dimensions of health are:

- *Physical* – mechanistic functioning of the body.
- *Mental* – the ability to think clearly and coherently.
- *Emotional* – the ability to recognize and express emotions such as fear, joy, grief and anger, including the ability to cope with factors such as stress or anxiety.
- *Social* – the ability to develop and maintain relationships with others, including one's family, peers and other members of society.
- *Spiritual* – personal values and principles, including religious beliefs and practices.
- *Societal* – an individual's health is affected by everything surrounding him/her, including aspects such as employment prospects, facilities for health care, transport, as well as politics and social policies at a local and national level.

An individual's state of health or ill-health is the result of the impact or influence of elements within one or more of these dimensions. Figure 2.2

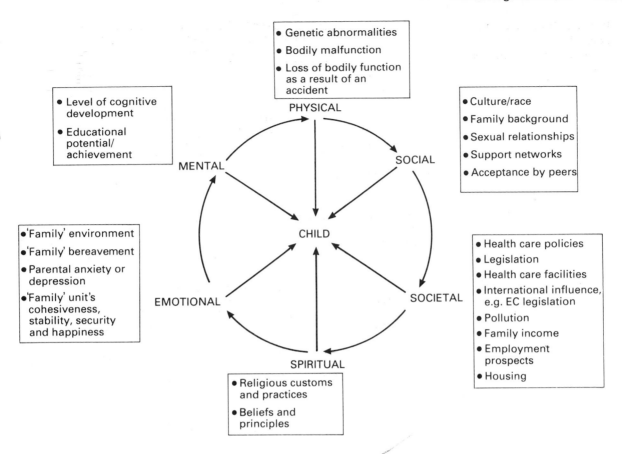

Fig. 2.2 The interrelationships between the dimensions and factors that may influence health.

highlights the interrelationships between the dimensions and factors which may influence one's health.

The child and family
It is acknowledged that the child is a unique individual with his/her own needs. However, the child constantly interacts with and forms part of a complex family unit and wider community. The child is influenced by factors affecting the family unit and it is recognized that the child can only function to his/her full potential within a stable family relationship. Therefore the whole family is seen as clients, rather than just the child. The term 'family' extends to include the person(s) who matter the most to the child (Fig. 2.3). The family's autonomy should be maintained at all times in order to maintain its integrity and for the child to feel secure in an otherwise strange environment.

The environment
The well-being and health of the child and family unit is seen to be interdependent with the nature of their immediate and wider environment with

Fig. 2.3 The family circle/meaningful person(s).

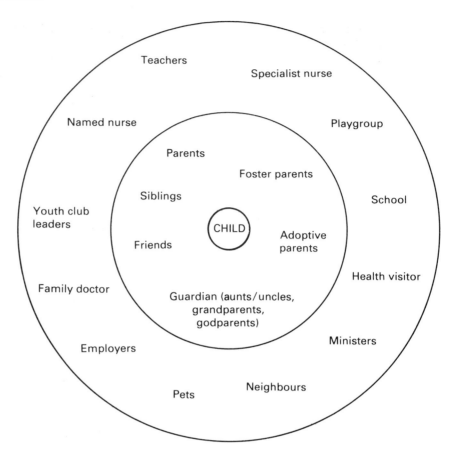

These are only examples and there may well be others depending upon each child's circumstances.

which they constantly interact. The environmental factors that influence the child and family are portrayed in Fig. 2.4. These have different levels of meaning and importance to each family unit. However, it should be noted that the family may change by developing or regressing, and therefore the importance or influence of these factors may also alter.

The Department of Health document *Welfare of Children and Young People in Hospital* states that children should, '. . . be admitted to hospital as in-patients only if appropriate care cannot be provided daily or in the community' [15]. This statement reinforces the belief that the best place for a child to be cared for is in their normal environment, in other words, in their home, cared for by their family carers, who are supported in doing so by appropriately skilled nurses. However, it must be noted that the 'normal' environment will vary for each individual child.

The nurse

Figure 2.5 demonstrates the relationships built and developed within a child and family focused approach to care. The three interlocking circles consist of:

Fig. 2.4 Environmental factors that influence the child and the family.

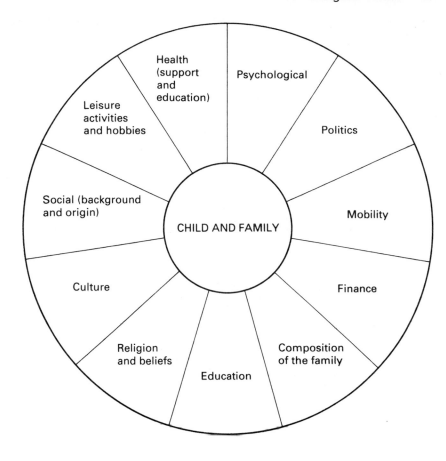

Fig. 2.5 The relationships within a caring approach centred on the child and family.

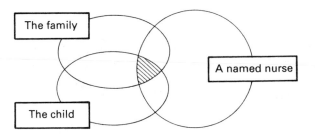

Whilst the overlapping areas highlight shared roles and responsibilities within the caring process, the shaded area indicates the potential involvement of members of *the multi-disciplinary team.*

● *The child* – an individual needing support to maintain optimum health or to achieve a comfortable and dignified death.

- *The family* – the child's normal or usual carers who need support to maintain a child's optimum health or to achieve a comfortable and dignified death.
- *The nurse* – a children's nurse who has the knowledge and skills to build an important relationship with the child and family. This nurse could be a primary, named or key nurse, associate nurse, specialist nurse or community nurse, who acts as a facilitator and supporter to enable the family to return the child to optimum health or to achieve a comfortable and dignified death. The nurse acts as the child and family's advocate, communicating between the child, family and the multi-disciplinary team.

The interrelationships between the four core elements

Figure 2.6 highlights the interrelationships and interdependence between the four core elements. The nurse acts as the main pivot, promoting self-care, independence and the maintenance of a family's integrity, as well as a sense of normality, whether the child is nursed within the community or hospital environment. This therefore highlights the importance of the child and family's nurse within the caring process.

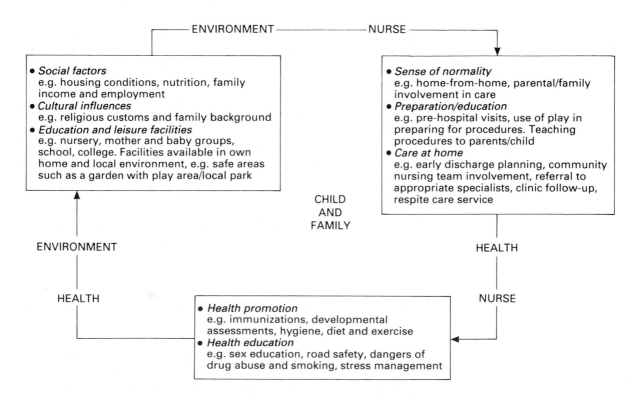

Fig. 2.6 The interrelationships between the four core elements.

The importance of the nurse's role within the caring process

Throughout the text pertaining to the model and its use in practice the named nurse, primary nurse or key worker is frequently mentioned. The role and relationship between this nurse and the child and family is of the utmost importance within this model of caring.

The hospital is a strange, frightening and daunting place for the child and family. This is especially so for the young child facing admission, who becomes exposed to unfamiliar surroundings, routine and strange faces. Those the child trusts, for various reasons may not be able to be with him/her continuously and therefore the whole experience can be extremely traumatic [62]. Primary nursing in conjunction with continuity in patient allocation by a named nurse is one way of reducing this trauma – the child has a 'special nurse', someone who knows his/her likes and dislikes, someone he/she can trust and rely on throughout the stay in hospital.

Most children admitted to the Nottingham Children's Unit are allocated a primary nurse. In some cases this is limited to long stay or frequent attenders. However, all children and families benefit from continuity in patient allocation, with care being provided by a named nurse. It is either the primary nurse or named nurse who assesses, plans, implements and reviews the child's care in conjunction with the child and family. The child and family are also involved in the selection of their primary nurse and receive an information sheet explaining that nurse's role (Table 2.6).

Although, support and advice from other nursing colleagues is always available within a primary nursing system, it is the primary nurse who has full authority within the decision-making process regarding the child's and family's care. The primary nurse is also responsible and accountable for ensuring that care prescribed is carried out and maintained; as well as for liaising with all members of the multi-disciplinary team and the communication of all relevant information to all those involved in the child's care [63–65].

As one nurse is responsible for the co-ordination of the caring process, there are obvious advantages in this system of organizing patient care. This nurse develops not only a special relationship with the child and family but also an indepth knowledge pertaining to their needs, thereby enabling the caring process to be appropriately geared towards meeting these needs. This includes ensuring that both the parents and child are involved in the decision-making process, that they are kept well informed, and that they are able to participate in the caring process as much as they wish to be involved.

The role of the ward manager or sister/charge nurse alters under a system of primary nursing. As the most senior nurse with continuing responsibility, the former's role is to:

- Facilitate a caring environment for patients, families and staff.
- Facilitate primary nursing and support those acting as primary nurses.
- Assist the primary nurse to develop his/her knowledge and skills so as to meet each child's and family's needs.

Table 2.6 Parent Information Sheet: primary nurse.

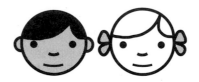

PARENT INFORMATION SHEET

PRIMARY NURSE

I am your primary nurse and will be the contact person for you and your family. I will help you and the doctors to plan .... care during this and subsequent admissions.

You can expect your primary nurse to:

Get to know you and your family.
Plan with you the nursing care to meet your child's needs.
Explain the plans to the associate nurse who will care for your child when your primary nurse is off-duty.
Tell you what to expect before tests or treatments.
Teach you about health care related to your child's illness.
Arrange follow-up and liaise with your health visitor/district nurse/social worker.

We need you to:

Tell your nurse what you want.
Keep your nurse informed about how you feel.
Tell your nurse if you have an idea or a preference about your child's nursing care.

If you have any questions about your child's stay please do not hesitate to ask me.

....
Primary nurse

- Act as a resource person within the team, offering guidance and information about aspects of care.
- Act as a role model by fulfilling the role of a primary nurse.

The model and the caring process

Figure 2.7 highlights the stages of the caring process, the key points of which include the following.

Fig. 2.7 The caring process: a continuous cycle.

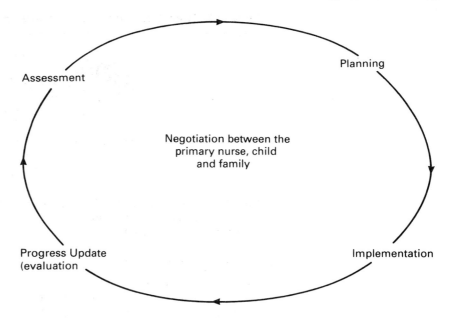

Assessment

Utilizing the Activities of Living (AoL) criteria, the nurse in conjunction with the child/family identifies the child's normal or usual level of independence and behaviour, physical and social development, and emotional state. Other factors within the child and family's immediate or wider environment are also taken into consideration. These include family circumstances, support networks, culture, prior experiences and knowledge about health and health care, beliefs, values, principles and preferences.

The assessment also includes identifying any deviation from the child's norm within each of the AoL. Incorporated into the AoL is an assessment of the child and family's ability to function independently with additional support, education and reassurance.

Planning

The plan of care is written in conjunction with the child and family according to those needs/problems previously identified as requiring intervention. Some needs/problems may not be those of the child or family but related to the child's treatment, for example, a need for isolation. The involvement of the multi-disciplinary team is therefore extremely important, along with an explanation to the child and family.

Care plans should be written in terms which the child and family can understand. They should be kept at the child's bedside along with other nursing records, the child and family being encouraged to read and assist with the completion of nursing records if they wish. Negotiated care that has been agreed with the child and family must be documented, acknowledging the child and family's right to alter their decision at any time. The plan should also incorporate and identify specific teaching needs and measures for support. The plan of care should reflect immediate and long-term needs/problems including those related to discharge and the potential for care to continue at home.

Implementation

This involves carrying out current care requirements as documented in the plan of care. Care may be required to be implemented or changed at any time. It also involves assisting, supporting, teaching and facilitating the child and the family to provide negotiated aspects of care. This includes recognizing that the child's family members also have needs/requirements, for example, see Maslow's Hierarchy of Needs [66].

Progress Update (evaluation)

In conjunction with the child and the family the nurse reassesses their needs and care requirements with a view to increasing their independence as well as facilitating discharge from hospital. The latter may include continued care within the community and the provision of respite support. The nurse records details in the Progress Update in conjunction with the child and his/her family so as to facilitate evaluation and the identification of any change in the plan of care that may be required.

The most crucial components of the above stages include:

● The importance of the initial assessment from which each individual child and family's problems/needs are identified (see Maslow's Hierarchy of Needs [66]).
● The factors that influence health and recovery.
● The concept of negotiated care.
● The active involvement of the child and family throughout the stages of assessment, planning, implementation and evaluation of progress.

However, it should be noted that this process involves not only obtaining information about the child and family, but also imparting information to them in order that they are able to participate fully and on an equal basis. This enables and facilitates the development of the child and family's knowledge and skills in relation to health and care delivery thereby assisting them to retain control and as much independence as possible by enabling them to attain a level of self-care.

The process is continuous, involving frequent re-assessments and the evaluation of progress. Adjustments should be made to the plan of care as necessary so as to meet additional needs/problems, or adaptation where applicable to meet those associated with continuing care at home.

Negotiated care

Negotiated care refers to a two-way process between the named nurse and the child, parents and family. It is based upon a relationship built upon mutual trust and respect, and within which each participant is equally valued. The negotiation process leads to a mutually agreed plan of care and level of participation in the delivery of that care, as well as an outcome and understanding that reflects each participant's capabilities and interests. However, the onus is upon the nurse to re-negotiate care and the involvement in care delivery according to the child's, parents' or family's wishes. This includes acknowledging their need for support at all times.

Fig. 2.8 A nurse negotiating care with a child and his father.

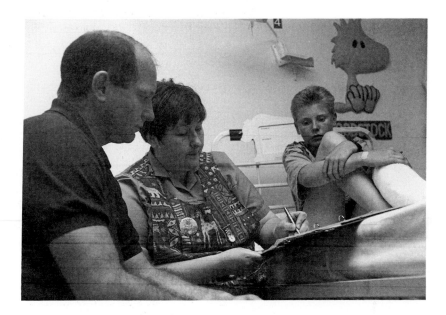

Negotiation and child/carer participation (Fig. 2.8) begins during the assessment stage, when the nurse obtains information concerning the child's normal or usual routine, level of physical and social development, behaviour patterns and psychological/emotional state, as well as their normal level of independence. Utilizing an adapted version of Roper, Logan and Tierney's [2] Activities of Living which facilitates the identification of any deviation from the child's norm, the nurse obtains the child's (depending upon their age, maturity and level of cognitive development or ability) and/or the parents' perception of the effect of the child's altered state upon each of the Activities of Living.

The Activities of Living (Table 2.7) that children and young people engage in within everyday life can be divided into: (1) those that are essential to sustain or maintain life; and (2) those that enhance the quality of an individual's life experience. Although some of the Activities of Living are not considered to be essential to sustain life, they can be regarded as necessary in order to maintain a complete state of health and well-being.

The language and terminology used in relation to the Activities of Living

Table 2.7 Activities of Living.

Breathing Eating and drinking Elimination Control of body temperature Mobility Sleep and comfort	Essential to sustain/ maintain life
Washing/care of skin/dressing Communication Play and learning (education/employment/social activities) Sexuality Emotional/spiritual	Related to the quality of life

incorporated within the Nottingham model reflect a child and young person's understanding and also relate specifically to those needs or activities that they engage in to live (with or without assistance from their usual carers and family). The level of independence is generally related to the child's developmental level. However, the latter in relation to one or more of the Activities of Living can be altered by the impact of factors such as: disability, physiological dysfunctioning, infection or an accident. Other factors, including social, cultural, environmental or personal preferences/ differences, also influence a child's basic needs or those normal pursuits or acts that they engage in to live.

The nature of each of the Activities of Living is fairly self-explanatory from the terms used. However, the Activity of Living 'emotional/spiritual' encompasses those pursuits, acts and needs related to enabling the child to achieve a dignified death. It also incorporates all aspects considered to be of paramount importance to the child's emotional or spiritual well-being, particularly in connection with relationships, as well as religious or cultural differences.

Within the general framework, those aspects related to sexuality are encompassed within other Activities of Living such as 'elimination', i.e. menstruation, or 'emotional/spiritual', i.e. relationships/behaviour or feelings related to one's body image. However, in the case of children with special needs, these are addressed under the Activity of Living of 'sexuality' itself.

During the admission period additional information such as family and social networks, as well as the influence of wider social and environmental factors which may affect a child's adaptation to a strange environment and thereby his/her recovery, are also noted. Other information that may impinge upon recovery or the child and family's health and well-being, such as a bereavement within the family unit or within their wider social community, is also requested.

Assessment also includes obtaining information regarding personal attributes, attitudes and beliefs held by a child and family, including those related to culture or religion, or those as a result of past experiences, perceptions and recollections of a previous admission to hospital. It is also important that the nurse ascertains the child and family's understanding of the diagnosis, symptoms, treatment or reason for admission to hospital (or need for continuation of care if discharged home), in order that any misunderstandings or misconceptions can be quickly corrected or further explanation given if required.

The aim is to obtain information so as to negotiate and incorporate measures into the plan of care that will maintain the child and family's equilibrium. This includes:

- The maintenance of as much normality as possible.
- The attainment of self-care and independence by the child or within the family unit.
- The promotion of adaptive responses by supporting and assisting the child and family to adapt to the strange and unfamiliar hospital environment, and the change in their circumstances.

The emphasis upon attaining self-care and independence, along with the focus upon the prevention of ill-health, health promotion and the maintenance of health, enables the model to be utilized within either the community or a hospital setting. However, the core emphasis is upon the maintenance or attainment of self-care and independence by the child and/or his/her family. Self-care has been defined as:

> '... a process whereby a lay person functions on his/her own behalf in health promotion and prevention and in disease detection and treatment.' [67]

In the case of paediatrics, self-care is interpreted as extending to the involvement of a child's family within the caring process. Thus the parents and family, as well as the child, should be involved in the assessment of needs, the planning of care, care delivery and the evaluation of the outcomes of that care. The nurse is seen as acting in a complementary way to enable the child and family to maintain their independence. This highlights the concept of negotiated care, with the nurse, child and family reaching a mutually agreed plan of care and agreement in relation to their level of participation in the delivery of that care. This involves an emphasis upon the nurse teaching, educating and supervizing the child and family about aspects of care, in order that they can reach a level of self-caring and retain as much independence as possible.

One cannot, however, overstress the need for the child and family's nurse to constantly consider the family's needs, as well as those of the child. The nurse should re-negotiate the level of their participation on a frequent basis, whilst ensuring that they feel not only supported when conducting the care they have agreed to provide, but also valued and prominent members of the team caring for the child.

The four stages of the caring process and the concept of negotiated care are presented in greater depth in Part 2, which incorporates an adapted version of guidelines related to the nursing records utilized within the Children's Unit in Nottingham.

Culture: its influence upon the caring process

Figure 2.9 highlights the fact that the caring process reflects and is influenced by attributes other than those influencing the relationship that develops between individual practitioners and a child and his/her family. The elements of the caring 'culture' can have a considerable impact upon not only the environment within which care is delivered but also the very nature of the caring process itself.

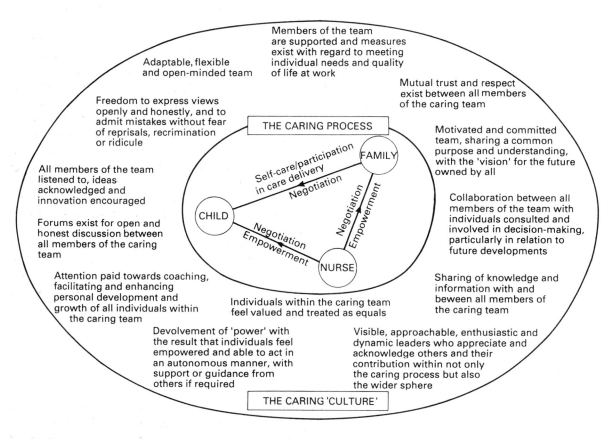

Fig. 2.9 The caring 'culture': the ethos of negotiation and 'working together' within the caring process.

The wider 'culture' or 'climate' of the organization in which care is delivered must exemplify and reflect the attributes, qualities and above all the attitudes that are valued and considered to be of paramount importance to facilitate the development of an equal partnership between the nurse and a child and family. Although collaboration and negotiation between and within the team are essential elements, the vital component is a 'culture' within which each member of the caring team feels valued, involved in decision-making and one in which all participants regard and treat each other with mutual trust and respect.

The creation of such a 'culture' lies with the leaders of the caring team, as ultimately it is they who set the tone and who shape attitudes within any organization. It is imperative that practitioners are led rather than managed or driven by superiors. Leaders must enable and facilitate individuals within the caring team to fulfil their potential and to develop and enhance practice. This includes guiding and motivating them towards a 'vision' and approach to care that is not only shared, but cultivated and owned by all participants.

A participative leadership style must therefore predominate. Leaders should share information and knowledge whilst also facilitating collaboration and the involvement of all members of the caring team in discussions regarding future developments and the direction of the organization. It is also essential that a flattened hierarchical structure exists, which reflects relationships built upon equality, mutual trust and respect, and within which individuals feel empowered to act in an autonomous manner within the caring process. The attitudes and approach of leaders must also demonstrate that they truly care for and care about each individual member of the caring team. Leaders must therefore be visible within the caring environment itself and openly acknowledge and express the value of each participant's contribution. It must be recognized that to achieve the optimum level of care and the desired approach within the caring process, time must be devoted to communicating with and providing support for individuals within the caring team. This also includes creating an environment that emphasizes the importance attached to meeting the needs of those involved in care provision.

It is only within a 'culture' and under conditions such as these that practitioners are able to develop a reciprocal relationship and partnership with a child and family based upon mutual trust and respect for each other's contribution, knowledge and capabilities, and within which each participant is willing to share knowledge, expertise and skills whilst also supporting each other.

Building an equal partnership

An equal partnership evolves as the child and family attain additional knowledge and caring skills, and develop competence and confidence in their abilities. Figure 2.10 highlights that the key is to empower the child and family, by sharing knowledge and information with them, enabling participation through teaching and education, and facilitating involvement through the provision of support and advice. This process begins during admission when the nurse recognizes the family's knowledge regarding the child and expresses the value of their participation in the child's care at whatever level the family choose. It is, however, essential that involvement in care is negotiated with the child and their family and re-negotiated on a

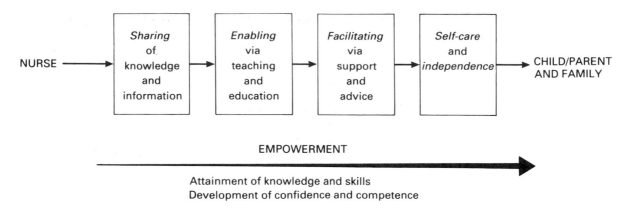

Fig. 2.10 Building an equal partnership within the caring process.

regular basis, so that they do not feel pressurized to undertake more than they truly wish or feel capable of at any point in time. Many of the factors inhibiting a child and family's participation and ultimately the achievement of self-care stem from:

●   The initial impact of the child's illness/admission to a strange and unfamiliar environment.
●   The child and family's perception of their ability to undertake aspects of their child's care, even that which is regarded as normal or routine (Table 2.8).

It is therefore essential that during the admission procedure the nurse adopts an approach that incorporates instilling a feeling of worth and confidence in the child and family's ability to undertake self-care.

Ultimately, the development of a true partnership between professionals and a child and family is affected by:

●   The attitude of the practitioner towards their inclusion within care delivery.
●   The willingness on the part of the nurse to share information, knowledge and skills.
●   The nurse's ability to educate, teach and support others within the caring process.

As previously highlighted the attitudes of practitioners and the approach to care are undoubtedly influenced and shaped by the relationships that exist within the caring team, as well as the ethos of the wider sphere and 'culture' within which care is delivered. If the latter reflects a highly hier-archical structure, the predominance of an authoritarian/directive approach and impersonal attitude, the caring process will undoubtedly be characterized by a paternalistic, depersonalized and dehumanizing approach to care. Such a scenario is likely to lead to a reluctance on the

Table 2.8 Factors influencing self-care and child/parent and family participation within the caring process.

Child

- Maturity
- Cognitive ability
- Developmental level
- State of health/severity of illness
- Desire to self-care
- Anxiety, fear and perception of own abilities

Child and family

- Child's normal state of health
- Severity of illness/condition
- Stage of hospitalization
- Anxiety, fear and perception of abilities
- Number of previous hospital admissions
- Previous level of skills and knowledge regarding health, health care and treatment
- Readiness and willingness to learn new skills
- Desire for knowledge, information and involvement in care delivery

Family

- Commitments
- Structure/composition
- Level of distress, stress and anxiety, and coping mechanisms/support networks
- Pressure within family to conform and participate/not participate

Nurse

- *Attitude* towards others and their caring skills/knowledge
- Value attached to parents'/carers' 'expert' knowledge about their child
- Ability to develop relationships built upon mutual trust and respect
- Willingness to share the 'power base' with the child/parent and family
- Communication and interpersonal skills
- Ability to educate, teach and support others within the caring process
- Ability to facilitate the development of additional skills within the family unit
- The 'culture' and structure of the organization

---

part of practitioners to share information, knowledge and skills with the child and family. This will therefore inhibit the development of an equal partnership within which the nurse, rather than acting as the primary care giver, adopts an educative, supportive and facilitative role, the latter being crucial in order to promote self-care and independence by the child and family. Thus, the nurse's role within the caring process is as follows:

- Friend
- Child and family advocate
- Information giver/provider
- Resource person
- Teacher/educator

- Facilitator
- Supporter
- Adviser
- Counsellor
- Co-ordinator

'The essence of the approach to care and the caring process lies within the hearts and minds of all those who participate . . . the values, qualities and attributes of which are influenced and reflected by the culture within which care is delivered.' (F. Smith)

A concluding statement

The Nottingham model is the culmination of many years' work and the development of innovative practice within the Children's Unit in Nottingham. However, the quote by Winston Churchill cited at the beginning of the book is extremely pertinent, for although the model as it is presented here reflects the values, beliefs and goals that guide nursing practice today, it should not be regarded as static. It is likely to be adapted, changed and modified as time passes and knowledge increases. Therefore, that which is portrayed here is only the end of the beginning and not the end itself.

Within the field of paediatrics (which many regard as a dynamic and forward-thinking speciality) there are undoubtedly many improvements and developments that as yet have not been made. As paediatric nurses, we should not be complacent with our achievements, but constantly strive to develop our practice further so that we continue to provide the best possible care not only for each child and young person, but also for their immediate and extended family. As Jolly [19] states:

'The challenge of paediatric nursing today is in meeting the needs of the whole child. This means not only attending to his physical care, but also paying attention to his thoughts, his feelings, and his need for his family.'

It is hoped therefore that the Nottingham model will inspire others to rethink and review their current practice, and to develop their own model of caring which will assist them in this process.

References

1. Orem, D.E. (1980) *Nursing Concepts of Practice*, 2nd ed. McGraw Hill, New York.
2. Roper, N., Logan, W. & Tierney, A. (1990) *The Elements of Nursing*, 3rd ed. Churchill Livingstone, Edinburgh.

3. *The United Nations Convention on the Rights of the Child* (1989) UNICEF, CRDU.
4. Rutter, M. (1982) *Maternal Deprivation Re-assessed.* Penguin, Harmondsworth.
5. Bowlby, J. (1952) *Maternal Care and Mental Health*, 2nd ed. World Health Organization, Geneva.
6. Bowlby, J. (1953) *Child Care and the Growth of Love.* Pelican, Harmondsworth.
7. Robertson, J. (1970) *Young Children in Hospital.* Tavistock, London.
8. Butler, N.R. & Golding, J. (1986) *From Birth to Five.* Pergamon Press, Oxford.
9. Douglas, J. (1993) *Psychology and Nursing Children.* Macmillan, London.
10. Muller, D.J., Harris, P.J., Wattley, L. & Taylor, J.D. (1992) *Nursing children: Psychology, Research and Practice*, 2nd ed. Chapman & Hall, London.
11. Department of Health (1991) *An Introduction to the Children Act 1989.* HMSO, London.
12. Department of Health (1990) *The Patient's Charter.* DOH, London.
13. Department of Health (1990) *Community Care Act.* HMSO, London.
14. Butler-Sloss, E. (1988) *Report of the Inquiry into Child Abuse in Cleveland 1987.* HMSO, London.
15. Department of Health (1991) *Welfare of Children and Young People in Hospital.* HMSO, London.
16. Audit Commission (1992) *Children First: A Study of Hospital Services.* HMSO, London.
17. Department of Health (1992) *The Children Act 1989: An Introductory Guide for the NHS.* HMSO, London.
18. Swanwick, M. & Barlow, S. (1993/4) A caring definition. *Child Health*, **1** (4), 137–41.
19. Jolly, J. (1981) *The Other Side of Paediatrics.* Macmillan, London.
20. Argyle, M. (1988) *Social Skills and Health.* Methuen, London.
21. Dobree, L. (1990) Pre-operative advice for patients. *Nursing Standard*, **4** (48), 28–30.
22. Boore, J. (1978) *Prescription for Recovery.* Royal College of Nursing, London.
23. Hayward, J. (1973) *Information: A Prescription Against Pain.* Royal College of Nursing, London.
24. Meng, A. & Zastowny, T. (1982) Preparation for hospitalisation: A stress innoculation training program for parents and children. *Maternal Child Nursing Journal*, **11**, 87–94.
25. Glasper, A. & Stradling, P. (1989) Preparing children for admission. *Paediatric Nursing*, **1** (5), 18–20.
26. Harris, P.J. (1979) *Children, Their Parents and Hospital: Consumer reactions to a short stay for elective surgery.* Unpublished PhD thesis, University of Nottingham.
27. Visintainer, M.A. & Wolfer, J.A. (1975) Psychological preparation for surgical patients: the effects on children and their parents' stress responses and adjustment. *Pediatrics*, **11** (56), 187–202.
28. Visintainer, M.A. & Wolfer, J.A. (1979) Pre-hospital psychological preparation for tonsillectomy patients: effects on children's and parents' adjustment'. *Pediatrics*, **64** (5), 646-55.
29. Hausen, B.D. & Evans, M.L. (1981) Preparing a child for procedures. *American Journal of Maternal/Child Nursing*, **6**, 392–7.

30. Stenbak, E. (1986) *Care of Children in Hospital.* World Health Organization, Geneva.
31. NAWCH (1985) *The Emotional Needs of Children Undergoing Surgery.* NAWCH, London.
32. Rodin, J. (1983) *Will this hurt?* Royal College of Nursing, London.
33. Stacey, M. (1970) *Hospitals, Children and their Families: The Report of a Pilot Study.* Routledge and Kegan Paul, London.
34. Vernon, D.T.A. (1965) *The psychological responses of children to hospitalisation and illness.* CC Thomas, Springfield, Illinois.
35. Harris, P.J. (1981) Children in Hospital – 1: Preparation of parents and their children for a planned hospital admission. *Nursing Times,* **77** (41), 1744–6.
36. Kiely, T. (1989) Preparing children for hospital. *Nursing,* **3** (33), 42–4.
37. While, A. & Crawford, J. (1992) Paediatric Day Surgery. *Nursing Times,* **88** (39), 43–5.
38. Report of the Committee on Child Health Services (1976) *Fit For the Future* (Court Report). HMSO, London.
39. Fradd, E. (1986) Learning about hospital. *Nursing Times,* **82** (3), 28–30.
40. Marriner, J. (1988) A children's tour. *Nursing Times,* **84** (40), 39–40.
41. Poster, E. (1983) Stress Immunisation: techniques to help children cope with hospitalisation. *Maternal Child Nursing Journal,* **12**, 119–34.
42. Melamed, B.G., Weinstein, D., Hawes, R. & Katin-Borland, M. (1975) Reduction of fear-related dental management problems using filmed modeling. *Journal of American Dental Association,* **90**, 822–6.
43. Melamed, B.G., Hawes, R., Heiby, E. & Glick, J. (1975) The use of filmed modeling to reduce unco-operative behaviour of children during dental treatment. *Journal of Dental Research,* **54**, 797–801.
44. Melamed, B.G., Yurcheson, R., Fleece, E.L., Hutcherson, S. & Hawes, R. (1978) Effects of film modeling on the reduction of anxiety-related behaviours in individuals varying in level of previous experience in the stress situation. *Journal of Consulting and Clinical Psychology,* **46** (6), 1357–67.
45. Bandura, A. & Jeffrey, R.W. (1973) Role of symbol coding and rehearsal process in observational learning. *Journal of Personality and Social Psychology,* **26** (1), 122–30.
46. Eiser, C. & Hauson, L. (1989) Preparing children for hospital: a school-based intervention. *Professional Nurse,* **4** (6), 297–300.
47. Ministry of Health (1959) *The Welfare of Children in Hospital* (Platt Report). HMSO, London.
48. Action for Sick Children (1991) *The Value of Play in Hospital.* Action for Sick Children, London.
49. NAWCH (1989) *Setting Standards for Children in Health Care.* NAWCH, London.
50. MacCarthy, D. (1979) *The Under Fives.* NAWCH, London.
51. Cross, C.A. & Swift, P.G.F. (1990) Observation and measurements of play activities on a paediatric ward. *Maternal and Child Health,* **15** (12), 354–61.
52. Delpo, E. & Frick, S. (1988) Play as a therapeutic modality. *Child Health Care,* **16**, 261.
53. Leese, D. (1989) My friend wiggly. *Paediatric Nursing,* **1** (3), 12–13.
54. Fradd, E. (1986) It's Child's Play. *Nursing Times,* **82** (41), 40–42.
55. NAWCH (1984) *Charter for Children in Hospital.* NAWCH, London.
56. Department of Health (1991) *The Children Act Series, Guidance and Regulations.* HMSO, London.
57. Sainsbury, C.P.Q., Gray, O.P., Cleary, J., Davies, M.M. & Rowlandson, P.H.

(1986) Care by Parents of their Children in Hospital. *Archives of Disease in Childhood*, **61**, 612–15.

58. Cleary, J., Gray, O.P., Hall, D., Rowlandson, P.H., Sainsbury, C.P.Q. & Davies, M.M. (1986) Parental involvement in the lives of children in hospital. *Archives of Disease in Childhood*, **61**, 779–87.
59. Jennings, K. (1986) Helping them face tomorrow. *Nursing Times*, **82**, 33–5.
60. Cooper, A. & Harpin, V. (eds) (1991) *This is Our Child*. Oxford University Press, Oxford.
61. World Health Organization (1948) *Constitution*. WHO, Geneva.
62. Jolly, J. (1989) The child's adaptation to hospital admission. *Nursing*, **3** (34), 40–42.
63. Pearson, A. (ed.) (1988) *Primary Nursing*. Chapman & Hall, London.
64. Wright, S. (1987) Patient-centred practice. *Nursing Times*, **83** (38), 24–7.
65. Manthey, M. (1986) *The Practice of Primary Nursing*. Blackwell Science, Oxford.
66. Maslow, A.H. (1954) *Motivation and Personality*. Harper & Row, New York.
67. Levin, L., Kratz, A. & Holst, E. (1979) *Self-care: Lay Initiatives in Health*. Prodist, New York.

Part 2

Using the Model in Practice

An Introduction to the Caring Process

The caring process involves the following four stages:

(1) Assessment of the child's and family's immediate, medium- and long-term needs.
(2) Planning the appropriate care for the child and family.
(3) Nursing action and intervention.
(4) Progress review and update.

The nursing records

The Children Act [1] published in 1989 suggests parents are usually the best people to bring up children. The emphasis within the caring process is upon assisting parents to adapt or increase their knowledge and skills so as to enable them to retain responsibility for meeting their child's emotional, social, developmental and health care needs. Whenever possible parents/ carers must be involved in decisions about their child. However, they must be given knowledge and information in an easily understandable language and format to enable them to do so on an equal basis with health care professionals. Children should be kept informed when decisions are made about their future. They should also be given the opportunity to participate in decision-making (depending upon their age, level of cognitive ability and maturity) concerning their health and welfare whenever possible.

The United Kingdom Central Council for Nursing, Midwifery and Health Visiting Code of Professional Conduct [2] maintains that registered nurses must, '. . . act at all times in such a manner as to . . . safeguard and promote the interests of individual patients and clients.' They are thereby accountable for their own practice.

These fundamental principles form the foundation of thinking when completing the nursing records. The nurse acts so as to promote the best interests of the child. However, it is acknowledged that the needs of the family must also be taken into account. The nursing records should therefore contain all the relevant information that may be required by the child and family's named nurse in order that the nurse is able to provide appropriate care which is geared towards meeting each individual child and family's needs.

The method of obtaining such information is based upon a systematic problem-solving approach, which involves:

- assessing the child and family's needs/problems;
- planning nursing action and intervention so as to meet those needs/ problems
- the implementation of care as planned in conjunction with the child and his/her family;
- a review of planned care with an update on progress [3].

The aim of the nursing records is to facilitate the recording of a child and family focused approach to care. The nursing records also incorporate those aspects that have been agreed as good practice in accordance with the Junior Monitor [4] and locally written standards (see the example below).

The nursing records are kept by each child's bedside. This facilitates a child and family focused approach to care, their participation within the caring process, as well as the sharing of information. The relevant records are completed or amended as and when care or needs change, rather than solely at the end of a shift. The emphasis is upon encouraging children and their families to participate not only in care-giving but also within care planning and the review process, the child and family being encouraged (if they wish) to participate in the updating and maintenance of all records including fluid balance or observation charts.

DRAFT

CHILDREN'S UNIT NOTTINGHAM

Standard Ref. No:_____   Achieve Standard by:_____

Topic: Independence & involvement of family/   Review Standard by:_____

carer_____   Signature of Senior Nurse Manager (Paeds):_____   Date:_____

Care Group: All patients on D35_____   Signature of Chief Nurse:_____   Date:_____

Standard Statement: All children on the ward should have current care to be given by parent/carer written in Child Action Column of their Care

Plan_____

CRITERIA

STRUCTURE	PROCESS	OUTCOME
Trained nurses who understand the Unit Philosophy of Care and have knowledge on the use of the nursing documentation.	(1) Explain to parent/carer within 2 hours of admission the Philosophy of Unit re parental involvement and negotiated care.	Parents/carer will have been given an explanation regarding the Philosophy of the Unit and parental involvement.
	(2) Explain to parents/carer care the child will require.	
	(3) Negotiate with the parents/carer which care they wish to give their child whilst in hospital.	The parent/carers' wish to be involved in their child's care will be recorded in the nursing documentation within two hours of admission.
Nursing Process documentation.	(4) Complete Care Plan and family/carer involvement in conjunction with the family.	Throughout the child's stay in hospital, the Care Plans will show an accurate record of parent/carer involvement.
Nursing Process guidelines.	(5) Show care plans to parent/carer and obtain signature to state they understand the care.	
	(6) Renegotiate the care each shift.	

References

1. Department of Health (1992) *The Children Act 1989: An Introductory Guide for the NHS*. HMSO, London.
2. The United Kingdom Central Council for Nursing, Midwifery and Health Visiting (1992) *Code of Professional Conduct*. UKCC, London.
3. Open University (1984) *A Systematic Approach to Nursing Care*. Open University Press, Milton Keynes.
4. Goldstone, L.A. & Galvin, J. (1987) *Junior Monitor: An Index of the Quality of Nursing Care for Children*. Newcastle-upon-Tyne Polytechnic Products, Newcastle-upon-Tyne.

Chapter 3
Assessment

As indicated in chapter 2, the primary or named nurse assesses the child's immediate physical and emotional needs on admission. This is then followed by a more detailed assessment of the child and family's needs/ problems.

Assessment consists of welcoming the child and family to hospital, and the introduction of their named nurse (or primary nurse) who then establishes a rapport with the child and family. Assessing the child and family's immediate needs on admission also involves obtaining an accurate history about the child prior to admission to hospital, as well as details related to the family unit. It should be noted that the assessment of a child and family's long-term needs also commences during this initial period, a fact that is clearly demonstrated by the History Sheets 1 and 2 (Figs 3.1 and 3.2). The whole process may not necessarily be completed immediately on admission, but may take up to several hours or even up to 24 hours depending upon the circumstances. The nurse must assess each individual child's condition and need for stabilization, as well as acknowledge the family's need for support and allow them time to adapt to the change in their environment and circumstances.

History Sheets 1 and 2

The required information is obtained from the child (depending upon age, maturity, cognitive level and ability) and his/her parents or carers. This process involves a two-way exchange of information. It provides the ideal opportunity for the nurse to establish a good rapport with the child and family. This facilitates the development of an equal partnership based upon mutual trust and respect. It should be acknowledged that the family has the best knowledge of the child and they *must* therefore be involved in the caring process from the outset, the nurse explaining to them the value of obtaining an indepth knowledge of their child, so as to facilitate the provision of effective care which promotes a sense of normality, whilst also meeting the child's needs.

Although adapted slightly for the purposes of this book, the following guidelines have been devised to assist nurses when utilizing the nursing records within the Children's Unit in Nottingham. They identify and highlight quite clearly the type of information that the nurse should obtain from the child and family. It should, however, be noted that they are only guidelines and should therefore be treated as such. There are no con-

CHILD'S HISTORY SHEET 1

WARD:			REG NO:
Family Name:	Date:	Time:	Family's perception of previous admission:
First Name:	Reason for admission:		
Likes to be called:			
Age:			
DOB:	Accompanied by:		
Birth weight:	Why do the parents think the child has		
Religion:	been admitted:		
Child's Address:			Parent(s) Carer(s) Resident: YES/NO
			Where:
Postcode:	Medical Diagnosis:		Likes to be known as:
			Do they wish to participate in the care of the child?:
Telephone No:			
Next of Kin:	What reason does the child give for		
Relationship to child:	this admission:		
Address if different from above:			Social Arrangements:
Telephone No:	Previous relevant history/admissions:		
Work: Home:			
With whom does the child reside:			
Relationship to Child:			Name and age of siblings:
Who has parental responsibility for this child?:			
Telephone number:			
Child's Nurse/Team:	Consultant:		

CHILD'S HISTORY SHEET 2

GP Address	Immunisation	Date or age administered:	Referrals made whilst in hospital, contact	Sign	Date
	Dip]	1st			
	Tet] Polio	2nd			
Tel No.	Pert]	3rd			
Health Visitor Address	Measles/Mumps/Rubella	YES/NO			
	Meningitis	YES/NO			
	Booster Dip. Tet. Polio (pre-school)	YES/NO			
Tel No.	BCG Age administered	....	Checklist for discharge info & referrals		
Health Centre Address	Booster Tet. & Polio School Leavers	YES/NO		Sign	Date
	Date of last Tetanus	....	Parent/child informed		
			Discharge advice sheet given		
Tel No.	Reason immunisations not given:		Equipment loaned		
Social Worker/other contacts					
Other information			Ward appt given to family		
			OPD appt given to family		
	Recent Contact with infectious diseases		Health Visitor informed		
			Community Nurse informed		
			Social Worker		
	Allergies		Doctor's Letter		

Ward Facilities - Tick box when explained to parents	Current medications & method of administration	Parent held records completed:		
Parents' Kitchen			Yes	
Parents' Sitting/Smoking Room			No	
Ward Kitchen			N/A	
Parent information board/file				
Parent shower/toilet facilities		Discharge weight		
Telephone		Medications		
Dining Room facilities				
Family Care Assistant				
Chaplaincy Department	Signature of nurse taking history: Date:			
Fire Regulations	Signature of nurse checking: Date:			
Facilities re-explained on ward transfer		Discharge Date Time		

Fig. 3.1 (facing page top) History Sheet 1.

Fig. 3.2 (facing page bottom) History Sheet 2.

straints, particularly in respect of individuality. Nurses may identify the need to obtain additional information which they consider to be crucial in order that they can provide effective care for a child and family.

History Sheet guidelines

The History Sheet(s) may be completed by any member of the nursing staff, the child or family if they wish. When this is completed by a student, auxiliary or health care assistant all information *must* be confirmed and countersigned by a trained nurse. If the History Sheets are not fully completed on admission (perhaps because it is not necessary or desirable) the nurse should sign each box separately and date it. The form should be fully completed as soon as possible. The nurse completing the form is required to check the whole sheet and sign it at the bottom. This process ensures that responsibility is taken for the accuracy of the whole sheet. If subsequent information becomes known at a later stage this addition *must* be signed, dated and the time of its inclusion on the History Sheet recorded. Any part of the History Sheet that is not relevant should have 'Not Applicable' or 'N/A' inserted into the appropriate box.

Copies of the nursing records are kept in the Children's Accident and Emergency Department and Children's Out-patient Department. This enables the history-taking process to begin whilst the child and family are waiting for transfer to the ward.

Personal details

Likes to be called   The child's choice (if possible) – nickname or full name.

Next-of-kin   Mr and Mrs Brown or Mike Brown and Lucy Brown.

Relationship to child   Could be parent, grandparent, foster parent, etc.

With whom does the child reside?   Could be mother, father, grandparents, foster parents. Include the father's/mother's legal access to visit the child.

Who has parental responsibility for the child?   Names and relationship, e.g. parents, mother only, social worker.

It should be noted that parental responsibility is not affected by parental separation. Parents who were or have been married to each other at or after the time of the child's conception each have parental responsibility for the child; otherwise the mother alone has parental responsibility [1]. Mothers and married parents only lose parental responsibility if their child is adopted [1]. Parents do not lose parental responsibility even when a child is admitted under a court order. Parental responsibility will be shared by the parents and the applicant for the court order.

Who can acquire parental responsibility?

- The unmarried father by a court order or a parental responsibility agreement with the mother without going to court.
- People other than parents by the private appointment of a guardian or an order of the court, e.g. foster parents via a residence order.
- Step parents [1].

Time, date and reason for admission

For legal reasons it is very important that the time of admission is documented. The reason for admission should be the *nursing reason* not the medical diagnosis, and should be written in language that is easily understandable and familiar to the family. For example: runny nose and cough; high temperature/'feels hot'; diarrhoea and vomiting.

Previous admissions

Information concerning past medical history should be obtained from the parents/carers and child. Any important details concerning past medical history can be checked with the medical notes. If there is inadequate space, a summary of the child's past medical history should be recorded on a Communication Sheet (see appropriate guidelines, chapter 6).

The family's perception of previous admission(s)

The feelings the family have about previous admissions and the parents' understanding of previous admissions should be recorded in this section.

Parent(s)/carers: like to be known as

For example, first names or more formal (Mr and Mrs).

Do they wish to participate in the care of the child?

An opportunity must be given for parents to choose their degree of participation in care. This section requires more than just an answer of 'yes' or 'no'; it necessitates that the nurse indicates what care the parents wish to participate in providing, for example, the child's usual care/nursing intervention, total patient care, or perhaps minimal care due to visiting difficulties. It is important that the nurse explains to the parents that although the Unit's philosophy is to encourage parents to participate in care, as well as to minimize the interruption of the child and carer relationship, the degree to which they wish to participate in the provision of their child's care is entirely of their choosing.

Social arrangements

Details recorded should be brief and informative, for example, any visiting or transport needs, who will visit, difficulties in arranging care for other children, or a need to see a social worker. Subjective and judgemental comments should *not* be made.

Other information

Once the History Sheet has been completed the nurse must ascertain from the parents/carers whether there is any other relevant information that may affect the child's stay in hospital, for example, the mother is pregnant, or a sibling that has died.

Ward facilities

The facilities available within the Nottingham Unit (see list on History Sheet 2 – Fig. 3.2) should be discussed and shown to families during the admission period. In order to ensure that *all* information has been given to the family, the nurse is required to tick each section when this has been completed.

Medication

Details of all medications, including dosage, frequency and time of last dose, must be recorded. Other information concerning the method of administration, i.e. spoon, syringe, tablet or elixir, and whether the child has anything else at the same time, e.g. orange juice, sweets, should also be recorded. Contraceptive medication should also be included in this section.

Immunizations

All parts of the immunization section should be completed. If immunizations have not been administered as per schedule, the reasons should be recorded.

Discharge section

This should include details pertaining to the discharge or transfer home of the child and family. The nurse is required to date and sign each aspect as these may be organized on an ongoing basis throughout the child and family's stay in hospital.

Referrals made whilst in hospital

Details concerning other referrals (to other members of the team or departments, e.g. the Child Development Unit, physiotherapist, dietician, chaplain, social worker, etc.), which may be made whilst the child is in hospital, are also recorded in this section. It is imperative that the name of the person to whom the child has been referred rather than just their title is clearly recorded. This enables other members of the team to contact the appropriate person if required.

Assessment Sheet – 'Gingerbread Man'

The aim of the Assessment Sheet (Fig. 3.3) is to gain a comprehensive outline of the child's usual routine and identify the Activities of Living that have altered due to the child's present condition or illness.

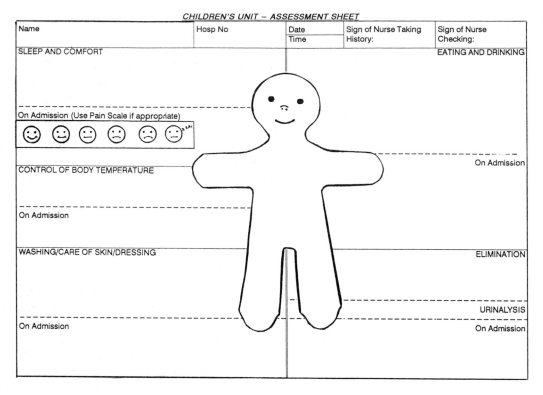

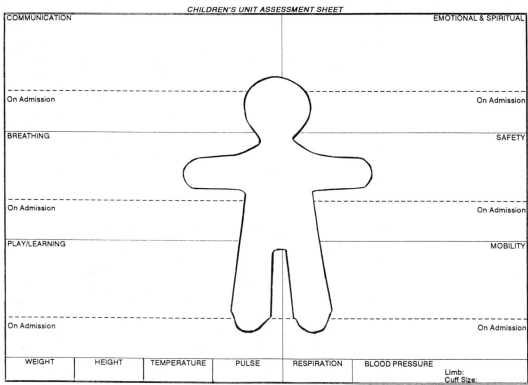

Fig. 3.3 (facing page) Assessment Sheet (Gingerbread Man).

Rationale

(1) To facilitate the identification of problems applicable to each child.

(2) To ensure the child's care is planned in conjunction with and at an appropriate level for the child and family, and is reflective of the child's normal routine as much as possible. It is important to remember that although the child's level of independence in relation to some of the Activities of Living may be modified by the child's condition, the child may, with encouragement, continue to be as independent as possible.

(3) Unless the child's normal routine is interrupted by illness, the information on the Assessment Sheet should be used to plan the child's daily care and should prevent unnecessarily long care plans, i.e. it is a working assessment sheet (see chapter 4).

Completing the Assessment Sheet

The initial recording of the child's usual activities should be undertaken within two hours of the child's admission. However, for various reasons it may be impossible to complete the assessment within this timescale. An example would be when a large number of children are admitted for a surgical list. In this instance the trained nurse within two hours of admission should ask the child and family if there are any special problems requiring immediate advice or attention, such as those associated with diabetes or epilepsy. This initial assessment must be documented, ensuring that the date and time are recorded on the Communication Sheet. This nurse must then complete the 'On Admission' assessment before going off-duty. The child's normal assessment may then be completed by the named nurse caring for the child on the next shift providing that the parents are resident. This assessment must always be completed before the parents/carers leave the ward.

It should be noted that even if the child's usual activities have not altered due to the child's present condition or reason for admission, the 'On Admission' assessment section still requires a statement regarding all of the Activities of Living that reflects the child's present health state and reaction to the admission.

Re-admission/internal transfer assessment

It is extremely important that the original assessment sheet is not added to or altered in any way. If a child is re-admitted within three months, a second Assessment Sheet is required. However, the original assessment of the child's usual Activities of Living can be rechecked with the family, with any changes being recorded in the appropriate section of the second Assessment Sheet. The child's condition on the subsequent admission must be recorded in the 'On Admission' section of the second Assessment Sheet. If a child is transferred from or to the Intensive Care Unit, a second 'On Admission' assessment must be undertaken as the child's condition will

Fig. 3.4 (facing page) Assessment Sheet for critical care areas.

have changed from that initially made on admission and therefore new needs or problems will be identified. The date, time and signature of the trained nurse must be recorded on this document.

The 'Gingerbread Man' figure

This can be used to:

- Identify the distribution of rashes/sores/bruises, e.g. Henoch-Schönlein purpura, and to monitor the spread of the rash.
- Facilitate a discussion between the nurse, child and family concerning the site of operations or to identify areas of pain.
- Allow the child to draw on and visualize an explanation concerning procedures particularly in relation to the anatomy and physiology associated with his/her condition or treatment, e.g. fingers, toes, hair as necessary, renal procedures or insertion of long lines, etc.

Assessment Sheet for critical care areas

The additional information on this sheet (Fig. 3.4) pertains to intensive care areas, where a rapid assessment of a child must be made due to the urgent nature of the admission or emergency situation. The content of the Assessment Sheet may be ticked or circled to facilitate the recording of all initial information regarding resuscitation and the critical condition of the child. However, the admitting nurse must record additional information before going off-duty. It is expected that an assessment of the child's usual Activities of Living should be obtained from the family within 24 hours of admission. If a child is transferred from a ward area to intensive care, an 'On Admission' assessment must be made and recorded on the Critical Care Assessment Sheet.

Assessment Sheet for children with special needs

Following an initial assessment and recording of the child's normal Activities of Living, this Assessment Sheet (Fig. 3.5) may be used for up to three months. However, an 'On Admission' assessment must be made for each Activity of Living and recorded, timed, dated and signed on each admission. The record of the child's normal Activities of Living must be checked with the family on each occasion and any changes recorded, dated, timed and signed.

Recognizing the needs of adolescents

Young people between the ages of 10 and 20 years are regarded as adolescents [2]. However, it should be noted that children up to the age of

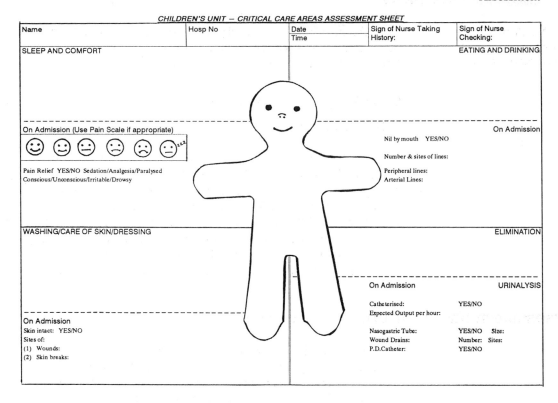

CHILDREN'S UNIT — CRITICAL CARE AREAS ASSESSMENT SHEET

Name	Hosp No	Date	Sign of Nurse Taking	Sign of Nurse
		Time	History:	Checking:

SLEEP AND COMFORT   EATING AND DRINKING

On Admission (Use Pain Scale if appropriate)   On Admission

Pain Relief YES/NO Sedation/Analgesia/Paralysed
Conscious/Unconscious/Irritable/Drowsy

Nil by mouth   YES/NO

Number & sites of lines:

Peripheral lines:
Arterial Lines:

WASHING/CARE OF SKIN/DRESSING   ELIMINATION

On Admission   URINALYSIS

On Admission
Skin intact: YES/NO
Sites of:
(1) Wounds:
(2) Skin breaks:

Catheterised: YES/NO
Expected Output per hour:

Nasogastric Tube: YES/NO   Size:
Wound Drains: Number: Sites:
P.D. Catheter: YES/NO

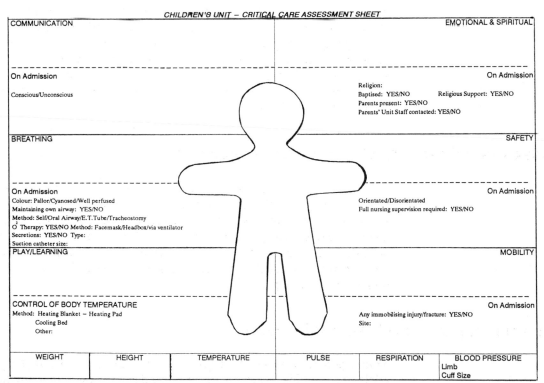

CHILDREN'S UNIT — CRITICAL CARE ASSESSMENT SHEET

COMMUNICATION   EMOTIONAL & SPIRITUAL

On Admission   On Admission

Conscious/Unconscious

Religion:
Baptised: YES/NO   Religious Support: YES/NO
Parents present: YES/NO
Parents' Unit Staff contacted: YES/NO

BREATHING   SAFETY

On Admission   On Admission
Colour: Pallor/Cyanosed/Well perfused
Maintaining own airway: YES/NO
Method: Self/Oral Airway/E.T.Tube/Tracheostomy
O_2 Therapy: YES/NO Method: Facemask/Headbox/via ventilator
Secretions: YES/NO Type:
Suction catheter size:

Orientated/Disorientated
Full nursing supervision required: YES/NO

PLAY/LEARNING   MOBILITY

CONTROL OF BODY TEMPERATURE   On Admission
Method: Heating Blanket — Heating Pad
         Cooling Bed
         Other:

Any immobilising injury/fracture: YES/NO
Site:

WEIGHT	HEIGHT	TEMPERATURE	PULSE	RESPIRATION	BLOOD PRESSURE Limb Cuff Size

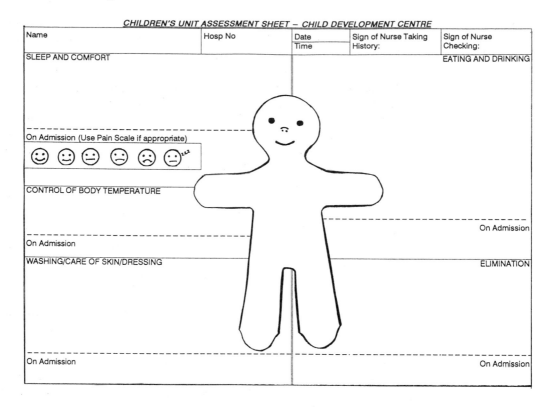

CHILDREN'S UNIT ASSESSMENT SHEET – CHILD DEVELOPMENT CENTRE

| Name | | Hosp No | Date | Sign of Nurse Taking | Sign of Nurse |
| | | | Time | History: | Checking: |

SLEEP AND COMFORT

EATING AND DRINKING

On Admission (Use Pain Scale if appropriate)

CONTROL OF BODY TEMPERATURE

On Admission

On Admission

WASHING/CARE OF SKIN/DRESSING

ELIMINATION

On Admission

On Admission

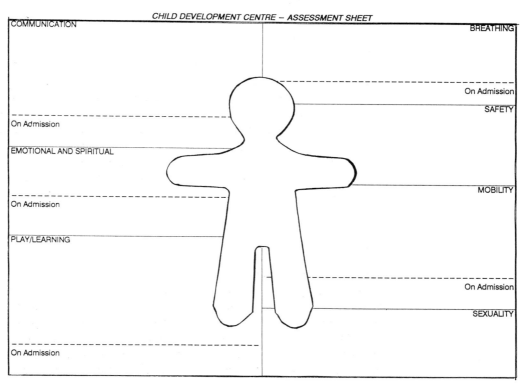

CHILD DEVELOPMENT CENTRE – ASSESSMENT SHEET

COMMUNICATION

BREATHING

On Admission

On Admission

SAFETY

EMOTIONAL AND SPIRITUAL

On Admission

MOBILITY

PLAY/LEARNING

On Admission

SEXUALITY

On Admission

Fig. 3.5 (facing page)
Assessment Sheet for
children with special
needs.

14 years and some 15- and 16-year-olds are cared for within the Children's Unit in Nottingham. Adolescence is viewed as the transition period 'between childhood and adulthood' [3], during which time the young person experiences many physical, intellectual, social and emotional changes. Adolescence, therefore, is a period of great change and adaptation, and is characterized by the young person's search for greater independence.

A number of reports [4–8], including the most recent Department of Health *Welfare of Children and Young People in Hospital* [9], recognize that adolescents are neither mini-adults nor big children, but a group of young people with their own special needs, and as such during a period of hospitalization require different facilities and approaches to care. Yet, in many instances adolescents continue to be admitted to either adult or children's wards which often do not provide an environment that caters for their needs [10–13]. Although their physical needs may be met, their emotional and social needs tend to be neglected. This is partly due to a lack of awareness amongst health care professionals concerning their needs, rights as individuals, their need for peer company, as well as independence and privacy.

Although the ideal would be to care for this age group in a specially-designed adolescent area this is not always feasible. In recognition of this, NAWCH (now known as Action For Sick Children) [8] and the Audit Commission [14] propose that young people up to the age of 18 years should be cared for under the auspices of paediatric units. Even within paediatric areas, many of the adolescent's needs, such as for privacy, can be met within existing facilities.

The adolescent's need for privacy

Adolescents are often easily embarrassed, especially in connection with their changing body image and it is therefore important to ensure privacy. In order to achieve this, many adolescents prefer to be nursed in single rooms rather than in a bay where their bed could be next to babies or young children. Although this may be very isolating and in many instances is not always feasible, it is often possible to ensure that children of the same age are nursed together in a bay. If at all possible adolescents should be involved in choosing their own bed, thereby increasing their self-esteem and to some extent allowing them a degree of control over their environment.

Promoting independence and self-care

Adolescence is characterized by a search for independence, increased decision-making and taking responsibility for one's own activities and future. Admission to hospital, however, may mean that the young person may lose this sense of independence and become dependent upon others. Yet, it is essential that he/she is encouraged to maintain as much independence as possible, by exerting some control over his/her environment and activities. The young person should be actively involved in all discussions and decisions regarding his/her health. Although, the young person's opinions and wishes must be respected, it is important to ensure that parents and families are also kept informed and involved in decision-making. Sibler [15] indicates that, 'Parental involvement is a recognized part of the optimal health care for adolescents.'

Essentially, parents continue to be responsible for the young person's welfare until he/she is 16 years of age, at which point the adolescent can override parental objections and can refuse treatment or give consent independently. The position of those under 16 years is less clear. However, the NHS Management Executive *Guide to Consent for Examination or Treatment* [16] states that:

'Where a child is seen alone, efforts should be made to persuade the child that his or her parents should be informed, except in circumstances where it is clearly not in the child's best interests to do so.'

Nevertheless, a legal decision in the House of Lords has indicated that the parents' right in respect of consent to treatment:

'. . . terminates if and when the child achieves a significant understanding and intelligence to enable him or her to understand fully what is proposed.' [17]

In other words, the youngster must fully understand the implications of what is being agreed or refused. The nurse's role, in conjunction with other health care professionals, is to provide information, to listen as the child expresses his/her fears and anxieties, and to assist and support the young person and his/her family whilst they make decisions concerning their future.

Self-care should be promoted by involving young people in the planning and delivery of their own care, as well as by enabling them to continue to maintain their normal routine and activities. The nurse acts as teacher and educator rather than total care-giver. Examples of promoting self-care, independence and self-esteem include:

- The provision of individual lockable medicine cabinets from which those aged 11 years and upwards can continue to be responsible for the administration of their own medication.
- Encouraging adolescents to keep their own fluid balance charts and to continue to carry out their own physiotherapy.
- Encouraging them to personalize their own room or bed area with posters of their choice.
- Encouraging them to bring in their own personal belongings, including computers, radios, cassettes and other items.

Promoting normal activities

Whilst in hospital the young person's choice of activities may be reduced as a result of the hospital environment and/or their illness. On admission it is important that the nurse identifies what the young person's usual activities are and incorporates these (even if in a modified version) into the plan of care. Although some restrictions may need to be imposed, it is imperative that the reasons for these are explained. Activities such as leaving the ward area, watching TV and bedtimes should be negotiated with adolescents thereby enabling them to continue to exert a degree of control over their lives.

Even if it is not possible to maintain their usual activities, boredom and frustration can be prevented by stimulating the development of other interests, such as art, crafts and computer games, as well as the continuation of their education which includes taking examinations such as GCSEs whilst in hospital. Hospital-based youth clubs and the provision of facilities which include noisy and quiet areas, along with access to simple tea and coffee making facilities, a TV, video, music centre and snooker facilities, prevent boredom and enable the young person to meet and mix with others of the same age. In many units adolescent groups have been set up, thereby promoting peer support.

The importance of maintaining peer group contact cannot be over emphasized, especially as maintaining links with school-friends and others undoubtedly assists with the adaptation process following discharge from hospital. Therefore, free visiting and encouraging the young person's friends and family to visit, as well as providing access to a telephone, are vitally important measures which enable the adolescent to retain links with the outside world.

In view of the different needs of the adolescent, the Nottingham Children's Unit has adopted the Charter for Care produced by NAWCH for adolescents [8] (Table 3.1). Although a separate adolescent area has not as

Table 3.1 Adolescents' Charter for Care (8).

---

(1) Adolescents should be nursed together in a separate unit which is furnished to meet their needs and is linked to the paediatric department.
(2) Adolescents should be cared for by appropriately trained staff who understand their physical and emotional needs and who respect their increasing need for independence.
(3) Adolescents need privacy and should be treated with sensitivity, honesty and tact at all times.
(4) Adolescents should have care that takes account of cultural and ethnic factors and the needs of those with a disability or chronic illness.
(5) Adolescents have the right to be informed about their condition and medical care and to participate in decisions about their treatment.
(6) Adolescents should be able to discuss their physical and emotional problems in confidence.
(7) Adolescents should be able to have their parents visit at any time and stay overnight if they wish.
(8) Adolescents should have every opportunity to maintain contact with family and friends.
(9) Adolescents need space for recreational activities and a quiet area for study.
(10) Adolescents should be provided with a written philosophy of the unit and agreed house rules with which they are expected to comply.

Fig. 3.6 (facing page) Assessment Sheet for adolescents. yet been commissioned, each ward and department has identified and improved facilities available for young people and a youth worker has been appointed to cater for their specific needs. The nursing records reflect the different needs of adolescents and include a specially designed Assessment Sheet for them.

Assessment Sheet for adolescents

The Adolescent Assessment Sheet (Fig. 3.6) is used for children eleven years old and over and has been adapted to meet their needs. Although it is very similar to the 'Gingerbread Man', it has some differences which are more appropriate to a young person's needs, e.g. hobbies/social activities and employment instead of play and learning. Adolescents are encouraged to complete this form with assistance from their primary or named nurse and to participate in decision-making about their own care and in the maintenance of their normal routine (Fig. 3.7).

Assessment Sheet guidelines

The following are *examples* of the kind of information that needs to be obtained from the child and/or the family. They are only examples and therefore they may not all be relevant to an individual child. The family may offer equally important information which is not included here. It is, however, important for the nurse to ascertain the child's degree of independence and the level of self-care with regard to each of the Activities of Living.

Sleep and comfort

Where the child sleeps:	Cot, bed, with parents, etc.
Time/patterns:	Rest in afternoon, sleep 19.00–06.00, needs a light on, sleeps on side or back.
Bedtime rituals:	Drink, story, dummy/toy or both, prayers.
Coverings:	Duvets, sheet only.
If wakes in the night/nightmares:	Action to be taken, give drink, change nappy, cuddle.
Comfort:	Special mascot (e.g. toy), blanket, cuddles. Medications (e.g. diamorphine elixir). Alternative measures – positioning, warm baths for pain. Recognition of pain level. If appropriate, let child use the pain rating scale [18] to indicate the level of pain on admission.

ASSESSMENT SHEET – ADOLESCENT

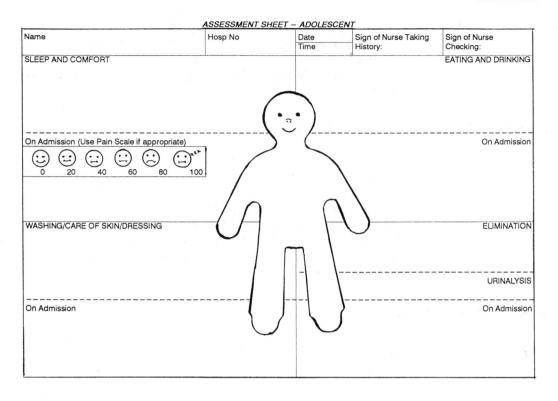

| Name | | Hosp No | Date | Sign of Nurse Taking | Sign of Nurse |
| | | | Time | History: | Checking: |

SLEEP AND COMFORT — EATING AND DRINKING

On Admission (Use Pain Scale if appropriate)

0   20   40   60   80   100

On Admission

WASHING/CARE OF SKIN/DRESSING — ELIMINATION

URINALYSIS

On Admission — On Admission

ASSESSMENT SHEET – ADOLESCENT

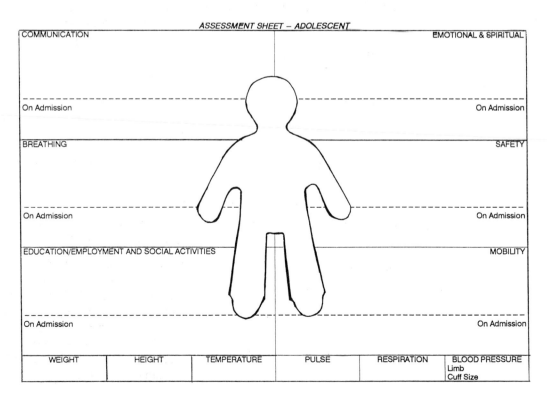

COMMUNICATION — EMOTIONAL & SPIRITUAL

On Admission — On Admission

BREATHING — SAFETY

On Admission — On Admission

EDUCATION/EMPLOYMENT AND SOCIAL ACTIVITIES — MOBILITY

On Admission — On Admission

| WEIGHT | HEIGHT | TEMPERATURE | PULSE | RESPIRATION | BLOOD PRESSURE Limb Cuff Size |

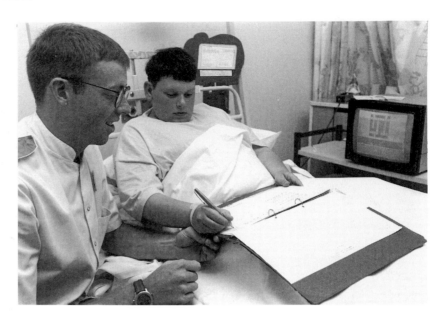

Fig. 3.7 An adolescent participating in decision-making about his own care.

Eating and drinking

Appetite:

Eats well/faddy eater. Takes 20 minutes to feed.

Portions:

Quantities/amounts – fluids/ scoops, etc.

Infant feeding/special feeding:

Breast/bottle – type of milk. Type of teat. Feeding times. Naso-gastric tube, gastronomy, intravenous feeding, etc.

Type of diet:

Tinned baby food, soft weaning diet, etc., according to age. Special/ halal, vegan/milk-free, diabetic exchanges/fat-free.

Likes/dislikes:

Dry cereals, no gravy, ketchup.

Utensils and independence:

Teacher beaker, knife, fork and spoon. Feeds self. Needs help. Uses fingers. Sterilization of utensils.

How the child is fed:

In arms, highchair, at table. How much assistance/supervision is needed.

Breathing

Any problems:

Wheezing, cough – productive/dry. Precipitating factors – exercise, pollen, at night. Colour (e.g. cyanosis). Physiotherapy – frequency. Nebulizers/inhalers – frequency, peak flows at home, average reading at home. Beneficial positions: tracheostomy – suction frequency, tube size/care. Speaking tube.

Smoking:

Quantity, when. Passive smoking.

Washing/care of skin/dressing

Routine/timing:

Bath times, frequency, assistance required.

Where washed:

Sink, baby bath, reference to privacy.

What is used:

Soap, Infacare, Oilatum, etc.

Special skin care:

Eczema, nappy rash. Creams/lotions.

Hair washing:

How often. Like/dislike – hair washing, shower head or bath.

Teeth:

When brushed, how often. Are they capped, loose? Does the child wear a brace?

Ability to dress self:

Put on clothes, cannot manage buttons yet.

Type of clothing:

Cotton only.

Special outfits:

Vests with pockets for long lines.

Temperature

Normal temperature control:

Extremities feeling hot/cold to touch, colour of hands and feet.

Coverings:

Gloves, bootees.

Response to raised temperature in the past:

'Grizzly', shivering episodes (rigor) or febrile convulsion.

| Present episode of high/low temperature | Duration, treatment given by parents, (e.g. 'sponging', space blanket, anti-pyretic medication, etc.). |
| Appearance of child on admission: | Clammy, sweating, flushed. |

Elimination

Toilet routine:	Special words used. Nappies, day and night/night only. Nappy size. Out of nappies but has accidents occasionally. Potty or toilet.
Frequency:	Twice a day, every nappy, plus once in night, etc.
Nature	Loose/tends to be constipated. Stream of urine.
Care of stomas/catheters:	Size and type of product used, care procedure, when usually given.
Menstruation:	Regular every 28 days, in middle of cycle, sanitation product used.

Communication

Sight:	Formal tests/infant follows light, bright objects, people. Glasses/ contact lenses – when worn. Blindness – hereditary, partial/total. Colour blindness. Injury, blurred vision, headache, intolerance to light.
Hearing:	Tests/turns or startles with noise/ voice. Hearing aids. Deafness – lip reads, etc. Grommets/glue ear, any treatment in progress. Reduced ability, ear injury, discharge/oozing.
Speech:	Language – English/Punjabi/Italian, vocalization level – babbles, small vocabulary. Speech difficulties – lisps, etc. Attends speech therapy. Sign language – type, Makerton, etc. Other methods of communication.

Mobility

Stage:

Rolling, lifting head, crawling, sitting up unaided, pulling up, walking with help, walking unaided. Indicate developmental level.

Aids:

Wheelchair, crutches, special boots. Exercise/physiotherapy. Positioning, use of splints, special chairs. Baby chairs, type. Use of baby walkers.

Safety

Level of supervision:

Hyperactive – cot sides/padding. Handicapped – helmets/harnesses. Baby/toddler – cot, reins. Devices for venous access – Hickman/Portacath, care routine. Convulsions – regularity and action taken.

Play and learning/education, employment and social activity for teenagers

Nursery, playschool, school, college and name.
Frequency of attendance, years 1st, 2nd, 3rd.
Hobbies/activities – water play, drawing, etc. Clubs – Brownies, Youth Club.
Developmental problems – extra schooling.
Any previous learning experience regarding hospitals.

Emotional/spiritual

Usual behaviour:

Lively, quick, extrovert, gregarious, loner.

Perception of self:

Body image.

Any recent stressful family event:

Changed school, moved house, new baby.

Teenagers: Change in relationships (e.g. within family), boyfriends, girlfriends and peer groups.

Religion: Christened, confirmed, barmitzvah. Other religious occasions of significance, e.g. Ramadan – fasting.
Any refusal of treatment on religious grounds.
Attendance at church, mosque, synagogue. Wishes to continue attendance whilst in hospital, Communion, Mass, etc.
Any special needs for the dying. Baptism, other rituals, contact Rabbi, etc. when relevant.

Assessing pain and discomfort

The accurate measurement and assessment of pain in children is a difficult area but one of paramount importance within the field of paediatrics. Research indicates that when a child's pain is identified and treated at an early stage, the child is not only more comfortable and more co-operative, but also the effects of hospitalization may be less than if the pain and discomfort go untreated for some time [19]. Yet many [20–24] indicate that there is a lack of awareness concerning a child's perception and experience of pain, and as a result the following misconceptions continue to prevail:

- Infants cannot feel pain because of immature nervous system.
- Children do not feel pain as much as adults.
- Narcotics cause respiratory depression and addiction.
- Active children are not in pain.
- Sleeping children cannot be in pain.
- A child engaged in play activities cannot be in pain.
- Children always tell the truth about pain.
- Injections are not painful.

What is pain?

There is no single definition of 'pain'. It is a highly complex, subjective, multi-dimensional and elusive phenomenon, which varies between individuals. Therefore, the word 'pain' has different meanings to each person and incorporates a wide variety of feelings, perceptions and experiences [20, 25–26]. McCaffery [27] indicates that, 'Pain is whatever the experiencing person says it is and exists whenever and wherever he says it does.'

This implies that an individual must be able to report not only when they are in pain but also where the pain is located. However, young children, either due to limited cognitive ability or limited verbal skills and developmental level, are not always able to interpret, understand or communicate this information to others. Other physiological, psychological, social, cultural and environmental factors such as birth order, gender, culture, social class and the influence of parents'/carers' attitudes, as well as past experiences, influence a child's experience of pain, their perception of pain and reaction to painful events [28–31]. Other significant factors are the attitudes, skills and knowledge of nurses in connection with the assessment and management of pain. Therefore, a lack of knowledge and skills, as well as understanding, concerning the manifestations of pain in children means that they often receive inadequate or ineffective pain relief.

A child's perception of pain

To a young child pain is often perceived as punishment for either real or imagined misdeeds. Feelings such as these are exacerbated by the fear and anxiety associated with hospitalization and the potential separation from parents/carers and family [20, 27, 31–33]. Many of these anxieties can be alleviated through:

- The provision of information and preparation for painful procedures/events, which is appropriately geared towards each child's level of development.
- The provision of a 'child-friendly' environment.
- The involvement of parents/carers and family in care provision, as well as the provision of facilities for them to remain with their child in hospital (see chapter 2).

Identifying a child in pain

In order to identify a child's level of pain and discomfort, paediatric nurses utilize a variety of means, including the observation of physiological signs and behavioural indicators [34] (Table 3.2), as well as asking the child about their pain utilizing pain assessment tools.

It is generally felt that children below the age of three years cannot identify the intensity, location and characteristics of the pain they experience. However, several studies [25, 35–38] indicate that children as young as 18 months can provide information about their pain. It appears that much is dependent upon the interpretation of verbalizations made by the child and the skills of the nurse making the assessment, as well as the use of language appropriate to the child's age when asking them about their feelings. Although reliance solely upon observation may be justified in the young infant, by utilizing appropriate and meaningful words according to the child's age and cognitive ability, the nurse may gain valuable and accurate information concerning a child's pain [39]. Often young children do not understand the word 'pain' but relate their feelings to words such as

Table 3.2 Physiological and behavioural indicators of pain.

Physiological indicators	Increased heart rate Raised blood pressure
Behavioural indicators	
● Vocalizations	Crying Moaning Screaming Whimpering Sobbing
● Facial expression	Grimacing Biting the lower lip
● Body tone/posture	Unusual posture Guarding Restless Reluctant to move Curled up on side
● Changes in behaviour	Aggressive (particularly amongst those with learning difficulties) Unusually quiet and withdrawn Increased clinging Irritable Lethargic Lying 'scared stiff'
● Changes in Activities of Living	Loss of appetite Disturbed sleep pattern

'hurt', 'sore', 'owie', 'hot', 'stings', 'upset' or 'frightened' [35–37]. Information such as this is obtained from the child or parents during completion of the Assessment Sheet.

Even if young children are unable to describe their pain, they are often able to accurately demonstrate 'where they hurt' on an outline of the body [23, 27]. The 'Gingerbread Man' incorporated into the nursing records can be used for this purpose. A pain rating scale is also incorporated into the Assessment Sheet of the nursing records, thereby enabling children to indicate their feelings on admission. This scale may also be utilized later to re-assess pain and discomfort, thereby determining the effectiveness of pain management. A working party within the Nottingham Children's Unit is at present investigating the assessment and management of pain, the aim of which is to devise a comprehensive and detailed pain assessment package suitable for use with children of all ages.

The pain rating scale

The use of a 'happy–sad faces' pain rating scale (Fig. 3.8) such as that produced by Wong and Baker [18] is easily understood by children from

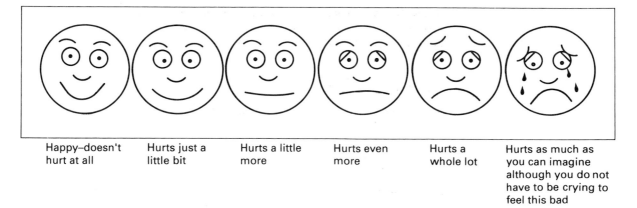

| Happy–doesn't hurt at all | Hurts just a little bit | Hurts a little more | Hurts even more | Hurts a whole lot | Hurts as much as you can imagine although you do not have to be crying to feel this bad |

Fig. 3.8 The pain rating scale.

three years of age, and combines a picture with a 0–100 numerical scale for use by older children. The faces depict increasing levels of pain and discomfort. The child chooses the one that reflects how he/she feels and represents the pain from 'no hurt' to 'the biggest hurt they have ever had'.

The use of a pain assessment tool such as this enhances the nurses' ability to assess and evaluate a child's pain, especially as its use often indicates that the nurses' perceptions of a child's pain are not always accurate [18, 24]. In many instances a child's behaviour or responses to questioning about the pain may not always be consistent with the level of pain or discomfort that the child is experiencing [21]. Some studies indicate that children may in fact deny that they are in pain so as to appear brave and 'in control' or to avoid being given an injection [21, 40].

In those instances where the child is unable to adequately communicate his/her feelings or denies pain and discomfort, the views of the parents are invaluable [33–36]. As it is they who know their child the best, they are often the best people to identify any changes in behaviour and to provide information concerning previous reactions to painful events, as well as coping strategies and the methods employed on previous occasions to alleviate pain. Price [39] and others [24, 41], however, indicate that due to stress levels and a lack of experience in such situations, many parents rely upon the skills of the nurse to identify when their child is or will be in pain. Nevertheless, it is imperative that they are involved not only in the assessment, but also in the planning of appropriate management, as well as in the evaluation of the effectiveness of pain control. This involvement leads to better pain control and results in an increase in self-esteem as the child and parents assume an active role and are able to exert a degree of control over what is happening to them.

Guidelines for the 'On Admission' section

The child's Activities of Living on admission or transfer may differ from his/her usual activities and it is these differences that should be recorded in this section. It is from this section that 'problems' requiring plans of care may be highlighted. *Examples* of the kind of information and observations that may be recorded in this section can be found below. If some of the child's Activities of Living are unchanged on admission 'No change' should be written in the appropriate 'On Admission' section with a statement reflecting the child's present health state and reaction to admission.

Sleep and comfort

Pain assessment: use pain rating scale – ask child if appropriate or assess.
Most comfortable position – lying, sitting.
Crying, awake, asleep.
Sleeping alone.
Medication – last dose.
Acceptable level of physical comfort.
Hot drinks, baths, etc.
Clothing – duvets.

Eating and drinking

Last meal, drink.
Describe any vomit, frequency.
Increased appetite, thirst.
Changes in level of independence.
State of mouth, tongue.
Diet and fluids willing to take.
Weight loss.
Nil by mouth.
Intravenous infusion, naso-gastric tube *in situ*, etc.

Breathing

Change in rate/pattern of breathing.
Noise, stridor, wheeze.
Action taken when apnoeic, colour/pallor, cyanosis.
Increased suction, nebulizers, etc. at home.
Increased oxygen therapy, etc.

Safety

Conscious level:

Orientated, disorientated.
Drowsy, rousable.
Dizzy, fainting.

Care of 'lines':

IVI, chest drain, monitor recording.
Permission for use of restrainers
(e.g. for cleft lip and palate).
Increase in convulsions.

Play and learning

Regression in academic work.
Attendance at school/nursery.
Interaction with peers.
Change in ability to concentrate.

Emotional/spiritual

Change in behaviour
Introvert/extrovert.
Awareness of condition/prognosis.
Spiritual support.
Parental support.
Other extenuating circumstances
(e.g. effect of a bad road traffic
accident or the death of a close
friend/relative).
Crying, irritable.
Ask the child how he/she feels.

Washing/care of skin/dressing

Physical anomalies: bruising, sores,
lacerations, dry skin, rashes.
Care of mouth, gums, teeth.
Change of dependence level in self-
care.

Temperature

Feels hot/cold, duration of
temperature, appearance.
Describe child's feelings.
Action taken to reduce temperature
before admission.
Clothing/blankets worn on arrival.

14. Audit Commission (1993) *Children First: A Study of Hospital Services.* HMSO, London.
15. Sibler, T.J. (1981) Ethical Considerations Concerning Adolescents and Their Parents. *Paediatric Ann.*, **10**, 47.
16. Department of Health/National Health Service Management Executive (1991) *A Guide to Consent for Examination or Treatment.* NHS Management Executive, London.
17. Mason, J.K. & McCall Smith, R.A. (1987) *Law and Medical Ethics*, 2nd ed. Butterworths, London.
18. Wong, D.L. & Baker, C.M. (1988) Pain in Children: Comparison of Assessment Scales. *Pediatric Nursing*, **14** (1), 9–17.
19. Smith, M. (1976) The Pre-schooler and Pain. In: *Current Practice in Paediatric Nursing* (eds P. Brandt, P. Chin & M. Smith). C.V. Mosby, St Louis.
20. Burr, S. (1987) Pain in Childhood. *Nursing*, **24**, 890–95.
21. Devine, T. (1990) Pain Management in Paediatric Oncology. *Paediatric Nursing*, **2** (7), 11–13.
22. Bradshaw, C. & Zeannah, P.D. (1986) Paediatric nurses' assessments of pain in children. *Journal of Pediatric Nursing*, **1** (5), 314–22.
23. Hawley, D.D. (1984) Post-operative pain in children: Misconceptions, descriptions, interventions. *Pediatric Nursing*, **10** (1), 20–23.
24. Buckingham, S. (1991) *An Exploratory Investigation into How Nurses Use Their Skills and Knowledge to Assess Post-operative Day Case Toddlers for Pain.* Unpublished thesis, B.ed (Hons) Nurse Education, Department of Community Health and Nursing Studies, South Bank Polytechnic, London.
25. Melzack, R. & Wall, P. (1982) *The Challenge of Pain.* Penguin, Harmondsworth.
26. Lutz, W.J. (1986) Helping hospitalised children and their parents cope with painful procedures. *Journal of Pediatric Nursing*, **1** (1), 24–32.
27. McCaffery, M. (1969) Brief episodes of pain in children. In: *Current Concepts in Clinical Nursing* (ed. B.S. Bergeson). C.V. Mosby, St Louis.
28. Mackey, D. & Jordan-Marsh, M. (1991) Innovative assessment of children's pain. *Journal of Emergency Nursing*, **17** (4), 250–51.
29. Broome, M.E. (1985) The child in pain: A model for assessment and intervention. *Critical Care Quarterly*, **8** (1), 47–55.
30. McGrath, P.A. (1990) *Pain in Children.* Guildford Press, New York.
31. Alder, S. (1990) Taking children at their word. *Professional Nurse*, **1** (6), 386–95.
32. Williams, J. (1987) Managing Paediatric Pain. *Nursing Times*, **83** (36), 36–9.
33. Gray, J. (1992) A painful experience. *Nursing Times*, **88** (25), 32–5.
34. McGrath, P.J. & Unruh, A.M. (1987) *Pain in Chiildren and Adolescents.* Elsevier, Oxford.
35. Eland, J.M. & Coy, J.A. (1990) Assessing pain in the critically-ill child. *American Association of Critical-care Nurses (Clinical Issues in Critical Care Nursing)*, **17** (6), 469–75.
36. McGrath, P.J. (1989) Evaluating a child's pain. *Journal of Pain and Symptom Management*, **4**, 198–214.
37. Jerrett, M. & Evans, K. (1986) Children's pain vocabulary. *Journal of Advanced Nursing*, **11**, 403–8.
38. Abu-Saad, H. & Holzeimmer, W.L. (1981) Measuring children's self-assessment of pain. *Issues in Comprehensive Pediatric Nursing*, **5**, 337–49.
39. Price, S. (1990) Pain: its experience, assessment and management in children. *Nursing Times*, **86** (9), 12–15.

40. Eland, J.M. & Anderson, J. (1977) The Experience of Pain in Children. In: *Pain: A Sourcebook for Nurses and Other Health Care Professionals* (ed. A.K. Jacox). Little, Brown & Co., Boston.
41. Copp, L.A. (1985) *Perspectives on Pain: Recent Advances in Nursing.* Churchill Livingstone, London.

Chapter 4
Planning Care

Care is planned in a systematic way using a problem-solving approach [1]. The Care Plan (Fig. 4.1) allows for one problem or need per sheet.

NURSING CARE PLAN

NAME			HOSPITAL NO.		AGE
ACTIVITY OF LIVING			PROBLEM/NEED		
DATE	TIME	NURSING ACTION	AMEND ACTION TIME, DATE AND SIGN	CHILD/PARENT ACTION	SIGN PARENT AND NURSE
				The signature of the parent indicates that this care plan has been negotiated	

Fig. 4.1 Nursing Care Plan.

Problems/needs

Everyone has needs, for example food and love, but when the child and family as a unit are unable to continue to meet these needs independently then the needs become 'problems'. It is then that nursing assistance is required in order that these problems can be met or overcome. For example, hygiene is not a problem to a baby as it is normal for a baby to receive full care from another person, but it may be a problem if an older child is unable to meet his/her usual hygiene needs in his/her usual way.

The nurse is able to determine deviations from the child's normal Activities of Living from the Assessment Sheet. However, a problem may arise if for example the child's condition or treatment represents a hazard to others as in the spread of infection/need for infection control or the hazards associated with chemotherapy. Nursing is concerned not only with problem solving but also with problem prevention. Therefore potential problems need to be identified as well as actual problems. Potential problems, however, should be realistic and relevant.

Whose problems are they? – the child's and in some cases both the child and family's. Problems experienced by the child must be described as such, except in the few instances when problems represent a hazard to others. The child's name must be used when identifying child-centred problems, e.g. John has difficulty in breathing. If the child has a long-standing problem or need which has become part of their normal routine, e.g. a long line *in situ* or a stoma or catheter, which is normally cared for by the parent or carer at home, the parent or carer's degree of participation in providing this care whilst in hospital must be re-negotiated on each admission.

The importance of using the Assessment Sheet (Gingerbread Man) (Fig. 3.3) as a working document *must* be recognized at all times as it contains information that enables the nurse to maintain the child's normal care. Problems that are identified must be amenable to nursing intervention. Problems should *not* be numbered as this may indicate priorities, which may not necessarily be entirely accurate, but Care Plan pages can be numbered if a problem index is used (see chapter 5). Care Plans are completed by trained nurses or student nurses under supervision, not nursing auxiliaries or health care assistants. However, any problems that the latter may identify must be discussed with the trained nurse with whom they are working.

A problem-solving approach to planning nursing care

A problem-solving approach is a system that effectively leads to an improvement or alleviation of a problem or need identified by the nurse in conjunction with the child or the child and family, and not a problem or need as perceived solely by the nurse. The Activity of Living appropriate to the problem is identified, e.g. breathing. The problem or need of the child is then also identified, e.g. coughing. The process consists of the following:

(1) Identification of the problem or need.
(2) Collection of information regarding the specific nature of the problem or need.
(3) Identification of a number of possible solutions.
(4) Decision as to which solutions are the most appropriate for the particular problem or needs.
(5) Prioritization of the solutions that will lead to the improvement or alleviation of the problem or need, and incorporation into a plan of care.
(6) Implementation of the plan of care.
(7) Evaluation of the impact or outcome of the plan of care.

It should be noted that *all* communication, including the identification of problems, must be written in a language that the child and family can easily understand. Jargon must not be used and medical terminology should be avoided unless the child and family have a full understanding of its meaning. Abbreviations should also be kept to a minimum, with a key included for those utilized, so that everyone is able to understand what is written.

Care Plans

The Care Plan is used in order to communicate the care required by a child to the nurse, his/her family and to other members of the care team. Care Plans should always be used in conjunction with the Assessment Sheet that identifies the child's usual routine or care. It should be noted that the Care Plan is a legal document, as it is the sole record of nursing care given to the child.

Care is planned using all available information, i.e. information from the History Sheets, Assessment Sheet, relevant charts, as well as further information obtained during discussions with the child and family. Throughout the process of identifying the problems or needs and planning care, the nurse should work in partnership with the child and family. It is also the nurse's responsibility to ensure that the family understands why they are encouraged to participate in the care provision for their child, and to give them the opportunity to choose the extent of their involvement.

Involving parents/carers and families in the caring process

Admission to hospital is a frightening experience for the young child who becomes exposed to strange surroundings, routines and unfamiliar faces. The whole experience can be extremely traumatic and can have long-lasting effects in terms of the child's development and normal functioning. Numerous studies clearly demonstrate the far-reaching psychological effects a period of hospitalization can have upon a young child [2–8]. These often extend into adulthood and affect future relationships, as well as employment prospects.

Although preparation for admission to hospital (see chapter 2), as well as the provision of a 'child-friendly' environment which meets play and educational needs, may go some way towards reducing the detrimental psychological effects of a period of hospitalization, the root cause of emotional disturbance is seen to be the direct result of separation from the child's parents and family [2–4]. As a result, numerous reports concerning the welfare of children in hospital, such as the Platt Report [9], the Court Report [10] and the Department of Health document *Welfare of Children and Young People in Hospital* [11] not only advocate the provision of a suitable environment but also stress the importance of:

- caring for the whole family;
- encouraging parents to remain with their child in hospital or to visit whenever they can; and
- involving parents in the delivery of care, as well as in the decision-making process concerning their child's care and treatment.

The importance of the presence of parents/carers

There is a wealth of research and literature that indicates that the presence of a parent or another family-member during a period of hospitalization substantially reduces the emotional trauma experienced by a child. They offer not only security but also continuity in an otherwise strange and unfamiliar environment [12–16]. Numerous studies indicate that their presence enables a child to cope with painful or frightening procedures, such as the taking of blood or induction of anaesthesia [17–21]. However, although parents are often the best people to prepare a child for admission or procedures, they often lack the information required to do so (see chapter 2).

Care by parents

As parents normally care for the child when he/she is sick at home, they are regarded as the child's natural care-givers [11, 22–23]. Sainsbury *et al.* [12] reiterate this, indicating that:

> '. . . the child's need for his parent is greatest when he is ill, and the sicker he is the more constantly he requires his parent.'

Therefore, encouraging parents and carers to participate in care delivery is extremely important, especially as this has been found to not only reduce anxiety and stress amongst the child and family, but also aid adaptation to the hospital environment, which in itself leads to speedier recoveries and shorter hospital stays [12, 24–27]. Involving parents and carers in the delivery of care also leads to less cross-infection, as well as better health education which leads to improved child-care at home and thereby decreases the likelihood of readmission [25–29]. Sainsbury *et al.* [12] indicate that the whole family benefit from the increase in knowledge concerning health and illness which is gained during participation in the care delivery process.

In the USA the importance of encouraging parents to participate in the delivery of care was first recognized when 'care by parent units' began to evolve initially as a means to reduce the cost of hospital stays. Although parents within these units undertake their child's total nursing care, it has become increasingly apparent over recent years that nursing presence is vital in order to alleviate anxiety, provide support and ensure better health education [30]. Parents or carers know the child best and have a wealth of knowledge concerning the child's needs. It is increasingly being recognized that they are the experts concerning their child and should therefore be actively involved in the planning of care, as well as in its delivery [31–34]. As a result, most paediatric nurses today recognize the importance of developing a partnership with the child's parents and family in order to provide care that is appropriately geared towards each individual child's needs [31–37].

Involving children, parents and other members of the family in care planning, care provision and in the decision-making process, not only enhances their self-esteem, but also increases satisfaction and enables them to maintain a degree of independence and control over what is happening to them or to their child [38]. Involvement in care delivery also promotes good relationships and better communication between professionals, parents and families.

Sainsbury *et al.* [12] indicate that many parents prefer to be actively involved in the delivery of care to their child rather than to be 'just resident' (Fig. 4.2). However, Jennings [23] indicates that there are different levels of participation in care delivery and therefore parents should be given the choice concerning the level of their involvement. Whilst some parents may wish to be solely involved with their child's normal care, others may wish to take a more active role and exert more control over their child's recovery. Therefore, participation in care delivery can vary from performing normal child-care and the recording of vital signs, as well as the administration of oral medication, to much more complex procedures, such as tracheostomy care or the administration of intravenous fluids or drugs.

Fig. 4.2 Parental participation in care delivery.

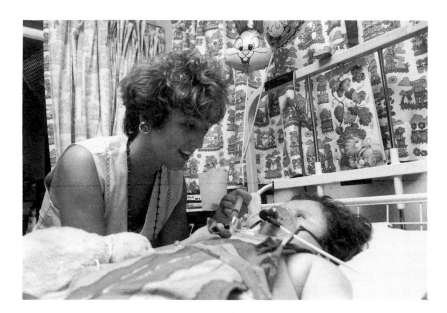

However, Knafi *et al.* [39] indicate that parents often receive little or no explanation concerning their participation in care delivery, and as a result assumptions are often made that they wish to be involved. Consequently, those who do not wish to participate, or are unable to do so, feel guilty and undermined. In this respect, many professionals fail to acknowledge parents' other commitments or preferences by not offering them the choice concerning their level of involvement within the caring process.

Evidence exists that indicates that professionals not only fail to offer a choice in participation but also undervalue the capabilities of parents. Several studies [12–13, 25] suggest that, providing parents have been given the opportunity to learn the techniques, most are perfectly capable of performing a wide range of quite complex tasks in addition to their child's normal care. Webb *et al.* [40] indicate that most parents are keen to do far more than nursing staff feel they are capable of. Parents may not always be given the opportunity to learn to perform the more complex tasks, even if they are willing to do so. In this respect many professionals pay only lip-service to involving parents and families in the planning of care and care delivery, as well as in the decision-making process.

Some professionals fail to treat parents as equal partners, and fail to fully appreciate their capabilities or respect the value of their role in caring for their child [22, 34, 37]. This can be partly explained by the fact that many nurses feel threatened by parents who not only possess a greater indepth knowledge concerning their child's treatment and care, but also are perhaps more adept at performing quite complex procedures. Therefore, involving parents in the caring process necessitates a change in attitude amongst health-care professionals, and the creation of an environment within which all participants receive recognition of their capabilities and feel equally respected and valued [41–42].

Yet, parents, during what they see as periods of staff shortage, often indicate that they are given too much responsibility, without adequate explanation, preparation or support. Several studies [25–27] indicate that it is the provision of supervision and support that leads to the reduction of anxiety and increased satisfaction amongst parents when they are involved in care delivery. A lack of support results in feelings of being undervalued, abandoned, exploited and abused. The provision of adequate supervision and support is therefore seen as vital to the success of parental participation in the delivery of care [34–37].

As parental involvement in the delivery of care increases, the nurse's role within paediatrics is changing from one of total care provider to facilitator, educator, supervisor and supporter [42–44]. However, it appears that some nurses fail to fully appreciate a parent's need for support irrespective of their level of participation in the delivery of care [34]. Yet, this must be acknowledged by all those involved in caring for the child and family, thereby ensuring that their stay in hospital is as untraumatic as possible.

The philosophy of the Nottingham Children's Unit (see chapter 2) recognizes the importance of involving the child, parents and family in the planning of care, care delivery and decision-making. However, the need to be flexible is also recognized, and the level of participation must be discussed and negotiated on an individual basis. The degree of parent/carer participation is discussed and negotiated on each admission, as well as on a daily basis, thereby giving them the opportunity to 'opt in' or 'opt out' of care provision as they wish. Negotiating the degree of participation in this way prevents parents from feeling abused and exploited, and acknowledges the fact that they are valued as equal partners within the caring process.

Case study 1
Jimmy Bradshaw: involving parents in the planning of care

The following case study demonstrates the application of the Nottingham model and highlights the parents'/carers' involvement in the planning of care, as well as the concept of negotiated care (see chapters 2 and 5).

Jimmy Bradshaw, an 18-month-old child, was admitted to Arnold Ward following a febrile convulsion. He was accompanied by his parents Clare and Tom Bradshaw. Staff nurse Sarah Jones greeted them on arrival at the ward. Sarah was to look after Jimmy during his stay in hospital.

Sarah, utilizing a systematic problem-solving approach, completed the History Sheet(s), assessed Jimmy's needs and planned his care in conjunction with Clare and Tom. The completed History Sheet(s) (Figs 4.3 and 4.4) demonstrate the commitment to care being centred on the family as well as the child. Examples include the sections relating to:

- Offering the opportunity for Jimmy's parents to be resident with him, providing the facilities to enable them to remain by his bedside or reside in the parents' unit.
- Encouraging Jimmy's parents to participate in caring for Jimmy during his stay in hospital. This particular section indicates that Jimmy's mother expressed the desire not only to be involved in the provision of his normal care but also to participate in controlling Jimmy's temperature.
- Social arrangements – Sarah's concerns extended to other family members, especially to the care of Joseph (Jimmy's four-year-old brother).
- Ward facilities – Sarah had shown and explained the facilities available within the Unit to Jimmy's parents.

WARD: ARNOLD	*CHILD'S HISTORY SHEET 1*	REG NO: 637292
Family Name: BRADSHAW	Date: 30/6/92 Time: 09:00	Family's perception of previous admission:
First Name: JAMES Likes to be called: 'Jimmy'	Reason for admission: HIGH TEMPERATURE HAD A 'FIT' AT 08:00	HAS NOT BEEN IN HOSPITAL BEFORE – AS A PATIENT NOR AS A VISITOR
Age: 18 MONTHS DOB: 2-1-91	Accompanied by: MOTHER & FATHER	
Birth weight: 7lb 6oz	Why do the parents think the child has been admitted:	
Religion: CHURCH OF ENGLAND	HAS HAD A HIGH TEMPERATURE FOR 24 HOURS & HAD A 'FIT' THIS MORNING	
Child's Address: 17 WINTHORP ROAD WOLLATON NOTTINGHAM Postcode: NG7 8PB		Parent(s) Carer(s) Resident: YES/~~NO~~ MUM Where: BY JIMMY'S COT Likes to be known as: CLARE
	Medical Diagnosis: FEBRILE CONVULSION	Do they wish to participate in the care of the child: YES – NORMAL CHILDCARE MUM WOULD LIKE TO PARTICIPATE IN CONTROLLING JIMMY'S TEMPERATURE
Telephone No: 297452		
Next of Kin: CLARE & TOM BRADSHAW Relationship to child: PARENTS Address if different from above: AS ABOVE	What reason does the child give for this admission: TOO YOUNG	Social Arrangements: MATERNAL GRANDMOTHER WILL CARE FOR JOSEPH AT HOME & WILL VISIT THE HOSPITAL WITH JOSEPH DURING THE DAY
Telephone No: Work: DAD 285313 Home: 297452	Previous relevant history/admissions:	DAD WILL VISIT AFTER WORK EACH DAY
With whom does the child reside: MOTHER, FATHER & JOSEPH	NO PREVIOUS MEDICAL PROBLEMS OR ADMISSIONS TO HOSPITAL	
Relationship to Child: PARENTS & BROTHER		Name and age of siblings:
Who has parental responsibility for this child?: PARENTS		JOSEPH – 4 YRS OLD
Telephone number: 297452		
Child's Nurse/Team: SARAH JONES	Consultant: DR MACINTOSH	

Fig. 4.3 Case study 1: History Sheet 1.

CHILD'S HISTORY SHEET 2					
GP DR T JONES Address WOLLATON HEALTH CENTRE STANLEY CRESENT NOTTINGHAM Tel No. 292717	Immunisation Dip] Tet] Polio Pert]	Date or age administered: 1st MARCH '91 2nd MAY '91 3rd AUGUST '91	Referrals made whilst in hospital, contact	Sign	Date
Health Visitor JOAN BURNELL Address WOLLATON HEALTH CENTRE STANLEY CRESENT NOTTINGHAM Tel No. 292717	Measles/Mumps/Rubella DUE NEXT WEEK YES/NO Meningitis YES/NO Booster Dip. Tet. Polio (pre-school) YES/NO BCG Age administered ....N/A...........		Checklist for discharge info & referrals		
Health Centre Address AS ABOVE Tel No.	Booster Tet. & Polio School Leavers YES/NO Date of last Tetanus .... Reason immunisations not given:			Sign	Date
			Parent/child informed Discharge advice sheet given Equipment loaned	S.A.JONES	30/6/92
Social Worker/other contacts NA			Ward appt given to family OPD appt given to family		
Other information NA	Recent Contact with infectious diseases NONE KNOWN		Health Visitor informed Community Nurse informed Social Worker		
	Allergies NONE KNOWN		Doctor's Letter		
Ward Facilities - Tick box when explained to parents	Current medications & method of administration CALPOL - 1 x 5ml tsp GIVEN EVERY 6 HOURS		Parent held records completed:		
Parents' Kitchen ✓ Parents' Sitting/Smoking Room ✓ Ward Kitchen ✓ Parent information board/file ✓ Parent shower/toilet facilities ✓ Telephone ✓ Dining Room facilities ✓	FOR THE LAST 24 HOURS. LAST DOSE GIVEN ON 30/6/92 AT 6AM SYRUP - ADMINISTERED VIA SPOON. LIKES A DRINK OF ORANGE WITH MEDICINE		Yes No N/A Discharge weight Medications		
Family Care Assistant ✓ Chaplaincy Department ✓ Fire Regulations ✓ Facilities re-explained on ward transfer	Signature of nurse taking history: Date: S.A. JONES 30/6/92 Signature of nurse checking: Date:		Discharge Date	Time	

Fig. 4.4 Case study 1: History Sheet 2.

The Assessment Sheet (Gingerbread Man) (Fig. 4.5), completed in conjunction with Jimmy's parents, identifies Jimmy's usual routine and care, and enables Sarah to determine deviations from his norm. These then become Jimmy's 'needs' or 'problems' which require a plan of care. One must remember that those Activities of Living that require intervention but which are due to Jimmy's stage of development represent his norm and therefore do not require a plan of care. His Assessment Sheet (Gingerbread Man) is therefore used as a working document in conjunction with the plan of care.

Figure 4.6 identifies the plan of care that has been devised by Sarah and Jimmy's parents in respect of controlling Jimmy's body temperature. Figures 4.7 and 4.8 respectively relate to the fact that Jimmy has not been eating and has been passing urine infrequently. Figure 4.9 identifies the plan of care in relation to a potential problem of Jimmy having further convulsions.

In respect of Jimmy's temperature, the care planning process involves:

(1) Identifying the problem or need – Jimmy has a high temperature.
(2) Identifying the possible solutions that will lead to an improvement or alleviation of the problem or need:

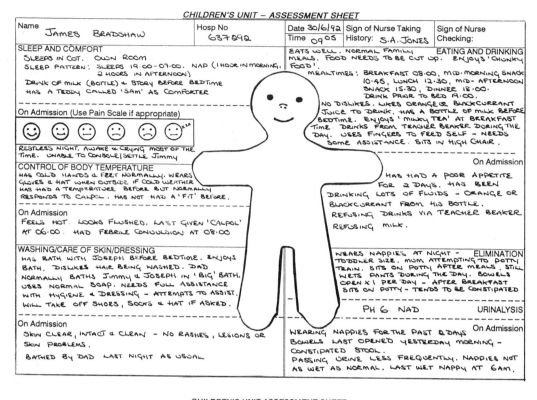

CHILDREN'S UNIT – ASSESSMENT SHEET

Name JAMES BRADSHAW	Hosp No 637092	Date 30/6/92	Sign of Nurse Taking History: S.A. JONES	Sign of Nurse Checking:
		Time 0905		

SLEEP AND COMFORT
SLEEPS IN COT. OWN ROOM
SLEEP PATTERN: SLEEPS 19.00 - 07.00. NAP (1 HOUR IN MORNING, 2 HOURS IN AFTERNOON)
DRINK OF MILK (BOTTLE) & STORY BEFORE BEDTIME
HAS A TEDDY CALLED 'SAM' AS COMFORTER

On Admission (Use Pain Scale if appropriate)

RESTLESS NIGHT. AWAKE & CRYING MOST OF THE TIME. UNABLE TO CONSOLE/SETTLE JIMMY

CONTROL OF BODY TEMPERATURE
HAS COLD HANDS & FEET NORMALLY. WEARS GLOVES & HAT WHEN OUTSIDE IF COLD WEATHER
HAS HAD A TEMPERATURE BEFORE BUT NORMALLY RESPONDS TO CALPOL. HAS NOT HAD A 'FIT' BEFORE.

On Admission
FEELS HOT. LOOKS FLUSHED. LAST GIVEN 'CALPOL' AT 06.00. HAD FEBRILE CONVULSION AT 08.00

WASHING/CARE OF SKIN/DRESSING
HAS BATH WITH JOSEPH BEFORE BEDTIME. ENJOYS BATH. DISLIKES HAIR BEING WASHED. DAD NORMALLY BATHS JIMMY & JOSEPH IN 'BIG' BATH. USES NORMAL SOAP. NEEDS FULL ASSISTANCE WITH HYGIENE & DRESSING - ATTEMPTS TO ASSIST. WILL TAKE OFF SHOES, SOCKS & HAT IF ASKED.

On Admission
SKIN CLEAR, INTACT & CLEAN - NO RASHES, LESIONS OR SKIN PROBLEMS.
BATHED BY DAD LAST NIGHT AS USUAL

EATING AND DRINKING
EATS WELL. NORMAL FAMILY MEALS. FOOD NEEDS TO BE CUT UP. ENJOYS 'CHUNKY' FOOD'.
MEALTIMES: BREAKFAST 08.00, MID-MORNING SNACK 10.45, LUNCH 12.30, MID-AFTERNOON SNACK 15.30, DINNER 18.00. DRINK PRIOR TO BED 19.00.
NO DISLIKES. LIKES ORANGE & BLACKCURRANT JUICE TO DRINK. HAS A BOTTLE OF MILK BEFORE BEDTIME. ENJOYS 'MILKY TEA' AT BREAKFAST TIME. DRINKS FROM TEACHER BEAKER DURING THE DAY. USES FINGERS TO FEED SELF - NEEDS SOME ASSISTANCE. SITS IN HIGH CHAIR.

On Admission
HAS HAD A POOR APPETITE FOR 2 DAYS. HAS BEEN DRINKING LOTS OF FLUIDS - ORANGE OR BLACKCURRANT FROM HIS BOTTLE. REFUSING DRINKS VIA TEACHER BEAKER. REFUSING MILK.

ELIMINATION
WEARS NAPPIES AT NIGHT - TODDLER SIZE. MUM ATTEMPTING TO POTTY TRAIN. SITS ON POTTY AFTER MEALS. STILL WETS PANTS DURING THE DAY. BOWELS OPEN X 1 PER DAY - AFTER BREAKFAST SITS ON POTTY - TENDS TO BE CONSTIPATED

URINALYSIS
PH 6 NAD

On Admission
WEARING NAPPIES FOR THE PAST 2 DAYS. BOWELS LAST OPENED YESTERDAY MORNING - CONSTIPATED STOOL.
PASSING URINE LESS FREQUENTLY. NAPPIES NOT AS WET AS NORMAL. LAST WET NAPPY AT 6AM.

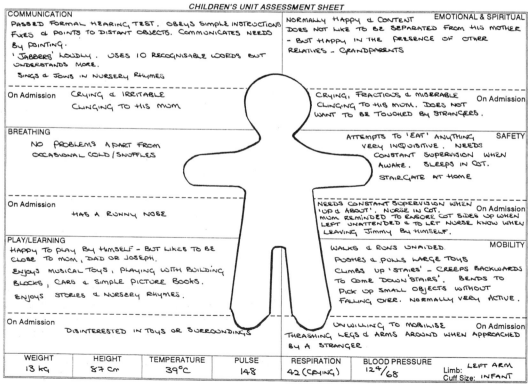

CHILDREN'S UNIT ASSESSMENT SHEET

COMMUNICATION
PASSED FORMAL HEARING TEST. OBEYS SIMPLE INSTRUCTIONS. FIXES & POINTS TO DISTANT OBJECTS. COMMUNICATES NEEDS BY POINTING.
'JABBERS' LOUDLY. USES 10 RECOGNISABLE WORDS BUT UNDERSTANDS MORE.
SINGS & JOINS IN NURSERY RHYMES

On Admission CRYING & IRRITABLE
CLINGING TO HIS MUM

BREATHING
NO PROBLEMS APART FROM OCCASIONAL COLD/SNUFFLES

On Admission
HAS A RUNNY NOSE

PLAY/LEARNING
HAPPY TO PLAY BY HIMSELF - BUT LIKES TO BE CLOSE TO MUM, DAD OR JOSEPH.
ENJOYS MUSICAL TOYS, PLAYING WITH BUILDING BLOCKS, CARS & SIMPLE PICTURE BOOKS.
ENJOYS STORIES & NURSERY RHYMES.

On Admission
DISINTERESTED IN TOYS OR SURROUNDINGS

EMOTIONAL & SPIRITUAL
NORMALLY HAPPY & CONTENT. DOES NOT LIKE TO BE SEPARATED FROM HIS MOTHER - BUT HAPPY IN THE PRESENCE OF OTHER RELATIVES - GRANDPARENTS

On Admission
CRYING, FRACTIOUS & MISERABLE. CLINGING TO HIS MUM. DOES NOT WANT TO BE TOUCHED BY STRANGERS.

SAFETY
ATTEMPTS TO 'EAT' ANYTHING. VERY INQUISITIVE. NEEDS CONSTANT SUPERVISION WHEN AWAKE. SLEEPS IN COT.
STAIRGATE AT HOME

On Admission
NEEDS CONSTANT SUPERVISION WHEN 'UP & ABOUT'. NURSE IN COT. MUM REMINDED TO ENSURE COT SIDES UP WHEN LEFT UNATTENDED & TO LET NURSE KNOW WHEN LEAVING JIMMY BY HIMSELF.

MOBILITY
WALKS & RUNS UNAIDED.
PUSHES & PULLS LARGE TOYS.
CLIMBS UP 'STAIRS' - CREEPS BACKWARDS TO COME DOWN 'STAIRS'. BENDS TO PICK UP SMALL OBJECTS WITHOUT FALLING OVER. NORMALLY VERY ACTIVE.

On Admission
UNWILLING TO MOBILISE. THRASHING LEGS & ARMS AROUND WHEN APPROACHED BY A STRANGER

WEIGHT	HEIGHT	TEMPERATURE	PULSE	RESPIRATION	BLOOD PRESSURE	
13 kg	87 cm	39°C	148	42 (CRYING)	124/68	Limb: LEFT ARM Cuff Size: INFANT

NURSING CARE PLAN

NAME	James Bradshaw		HOSPITAL NO. 637292		AGE 18/12

| ACTIVITY OF LIVING Control of Body Temperature | | | PROBLEM/NEED Jimmy has a High Temperature | | |

DATE	TIME	NURSING ACTION	AMEND ACTION TIME, DATE AND SIGN	CHILD/PARENT ACTION	SIGN PARENT AND NURSE
30/6/92	09-20				
		* Nurse in cool, loose clothing – as minimal amount as possible			
		* Record temperature every 2 hours		* Assist with recording Jimmy's temperature every 2 hours following instruction (during the day, at night only when awake)	
		* Administer paracetamol as prescribed & monitor effect			
		* Encourage cool fluids & record on fluid balance chart		* Mum to offer 60mls (2ozs) of fluid every 2 hours & to record fluid taken on fluid balance chart	—
		* Commence fan therapy			
		* Obtain a/throat swab	30/6/92 10-40 S.A. Jones		
		* Discuss parent/information leaflet re: control of body temperature/with Clare & Tom	30/6/92 13-00 S.A. Jones		
					C. Bradshaw
					S.A. Jones
				The signature of the parent indicates that this care plan has been negotiated	

Fig. 4.6 Case study 1: Nursing Care Plan – control of body temperature.

- reduce clothing
- give fan therapy
- administer prescribed anti-pyretics
- record temperature frequently
- encourage the intake of cool fluids
- open all windows (with precautions to ensure the child's safety).

(3) Deciding which of these measures are the most appropriate for Jimmy.
(4) Prioritizing the possible solutions:

- reduce clothing
- record temperature frequently
- administer prescribed anti-pyretics
- encourage the intake of cool fluids
- give fan therapy.

Figure 4.6 highlights the concept of negotiated care (see chapters 2 and 5). Clare (Jimmy's mother) expressed the desire to participate in controlling Jimmy's temperature (see Fig. 4.3 – History Sheet 1) and has agreed with Sarah that following instruction she will record Jimmy's temperature every two hours, as well as encourage him to take cold drinks, recording those consumed on his fluid balance chart.

In order for Clare and Tom to form an equal partnership with Sarah, the need for education or the imparting of knowledge/information to Clare and Tom has

Fig. 4.5 (facing page) Case Study 1: Assessment Sheet (Gingerbread Man).

NURSING CARE PLAN

NAME	JAMES BRADSHAW			HOSPITAL NO...... 637292		AGE 18/12

ACTIVITY OF LIVING ...EATING & DRINKING........ PROBLEM/NEED ..JIMMY HAS NOT BEEN EATING........

DATE	TIME	NURSING ACTION	AMEND ACTION TIME, DATE AND SIGN	CHILD/PARENT ACTION	SIGN PARENT AND NURSE
30/6/92	09-30				
		* WEIGH ON ADMISSION & THEN TWICE A WEEK (TUES & FRI)			
		* OFFER BLACKCURRANT / ORANGE JUICE VIA BOTTLE EVERY 2 HOURS		* CLARE TO OFFER 60mls (2oz) OF FLUID EVERY 2 HOURS	
		* OFFER SMALL AMOUNTS OF FAVOURITE FOODS & SNACKS AT JIMMY'S NORMAL MEALTIMES OR AS DESIRED		* CLARE TO ARRANGE TO HAVE JIMMY'S FAVOURITE DRINKS & 'FOODS' BROUGHT IN FROM HOME	
		* RECORD FLUID & DIET CONSUMED ON FLUID BALANCE CHART		* CLARE TO RECORD FLUID & DIET CONSUMED ON FLUID BALANCE CHART	
		* GIVE MOUTHCARE EVERY 2-4 HOURS OR AS REQUIRED IF FLUIDS NOT TAKEN		* FOLLOWING INSTRUCTION CLARE WILL GIVE MOUTHCARE AS REQUIRED & APPLY VASELINE TO JIMMY'S LIPS	
					C. BRADSHAW
					S.A. JONES

The signature of the parent indicates that this care plan has been negotiated

NURSING CARE PLAN

NAME	JAMES BRADSHAW			HOSPITAL NO...... 637292		AGE 18/12

ACTIVITY OF LIVING ......ELIMINATION............... PROBLEM/NEED ..JIMMY HAS BEEN HAVING FEWER WET NAPPIES

DATE	TIME	NURSING ACTION	AMEND ACTION TIME, DATE AND SIGN	CHILD/PARENT ACTION	SIGN PARENT AND NURSE
30/6/92	09-30				
		* OBTAIN CLEAN CATCH SAMPLE OF URINE	30/6/92 10.30 S.A. JONES	FOLLOWING INSTRUCTION CLARE WILL ASSIST TO 'CATCH' THE URINE SAMPLE	
		* WARD TEST URINE	30/6/92 10.30 S.A. JONES		
		* OBSERVE FOR SIGNS OF PAIN & DISCOMFORT WHEN PASSING URINE & REPORT TO MEDICAL STAFF		CLARE TO REPORT ANY ALTERATION FROM JIMMY'S NORMAL TO SARAH	
		* OBSERVE FOR ANY ALTERATION IN COLOUR OR ODOUR OF URINE & REPORT TO MEDICAL STAFF.			
		* RECORD NUMBER OF WET NAPPIES & INDICATE DEGREE OF 'WETNESS' ie. DAMP / VERY WET, ON FLUID BALANCE CHART. REPORT TO MEDICAL STAFF IF DECREASE IN URINE OUTPUT		CLARE TO RECORD WET NAPPIES ON FLUID BALANCE CHART.	
					C. BRADSHAW
					S.A. JONES

The signature of the parent indicates that this care plan has been negotiated

NURSING CARE PLAN

NAME	James Bradshaw		HOSPITAL NO. 637 292			AGE 18/12

ACTIVITY OF LIVING ... SAFETY .... PROBLEM/NEED ... Jimmy may have further convulsions

DATE	TIME	NURSING ACTION	AMEND ACTION TIME, DATE AND SIGN	CHILD/PARENT ACTION	SIGN PARENT AND NURSE
30/6/92	09.20	* Ensure that Jimmy is nursed near working oxygen & suction			
		* Discuss parent information leaflet re: course of action to be taken if Jimmy has a further convulsion	30/6/92 13.00 S.A.Jones		
		* Place Jimmy in the recovery position if he has a further convulsion & inform medical staff immediately		Clare to place Jimmy in recovery position & press emergency buzzer if he has a further febrile convulsion when she is with him	
				Clare to inform Sarah if she is leaving Jimmy alone in his cot – Sarah will then observe Jimmy more closely	
		* Administer anticonvulsant therapy as prescribed, monitor & record effect			
					C. Bradshaw
					S.A.Jones
				The signature of the parent indicates that this care plan has been negotiated	

Fig. 4.9 Case study 1: Nursing Care Plan – safety.

Fig. 4.7 (facing page top) Case study 1: Nursing Care Plan – eating and drinking.

Fig. 4.8 (facing page bottom) Case study 1: Nursing Care Plan – elimination.

been acknowledged. This is demonstrated by Fig. 4.9 which highlights that following a discussion with Sarah, Clare is aware of the course of action to take should Jimmy have a further convulsion. Clare has signed the Care Plans, acknowledging that this is a true record of the level of participation in Jimmy's care that she has agreed and negotiated with Sarah. Figures 4.10–4.13 indicate that Sarah has reviewed Jimmy's progress and the care that has been delivered to him as it has occurred, rather than purely at the end of her shift.

This case study highlights the key aspects of the Nottingham model – care being centred on the child and family and the concept of negotiated care.

NURSING CARE PLAN – PROGRESS UPDATE

NAME	James Bradshaw		HOSPITAL NO. 637 292	AGE 18/12
DATE	TIME	ACTIVITY OF LIVING CONTROL OF BODY TEMPERATURE	PROBLEM/NEED Jimmy has a high temperature	SIGN
30/6/92	10·40	Throat swab taken		S.A.Jones
	11·00	Temperature 38·6°C. Paracetamol given as prescribed. Fan therapy continues		S.A.Jones
	13·00	Parent information leaflet re: control of body temperature discussed with Clare & Tom.		S.A.Jones

Fig. 4.10 Case study 1: Progress Update – control of body temperature.

NURSING CARE PLAN – PROGRESS UPDATE

NAME .....James Bradshaw.....		HOSPITAL NO ....637292........	AGE ..18/12....	
DATE	TIME	ACTIVITY OF LIVING ..Eating & Drinking....PROBLEM/NEED ..Jimmy has not been eating..		SIGN
30/6/92	13·00	Small amounts of blackcurrant juice taken & tolerated. Refusing		
		diet		S.A.Jones

Fig. 4.11 Case study 1: Progress Update – eating and drinking.

NURSING CARE PLAN – PROGRESS UPDATE

NAME ..James Bradshaw.....		HOSPITAL NO ....637292........	AGE ..18/12....	
DATE	TIME	ACTIVITY OF LIVING ....Elimination....PROBLEM/NEED ..Jimmy has been having fewer wet nappies..		SIGN
30/6/92	10·30	Clean catch urine obtained		S.A.Jones

Fig. 4.12 Case study 1: Progress Update – elimination.

NURSING CARE PLAN – PROGRESS UPDATE

NAME ..James Bradshaw.....		HOSPITAL NO ....637292........	AGE ..18/12....	
DATE	TIME	ACTIVITY OF LIVING .....Safety....PROBLEM/NEED ..Jimmy may have further convulsions		SIGN
30/6/92	11·00	Parent information leaflet re: course of action to be taken if Jimmy		
		has further convulsions, discussed with parents. Recovery position		
		demonstrated & Clare & Tom shown the location of the emergency		
		buzzer		S.A.Jones
	13·00	No further convulsions		S.A.Jones

Fig. 4.13 Case study 1: Progress Update – safety.

References

1. Open University (1984) *A Systematic Approach to Nursing Care.* Open University Press, Milton Keynes.
2. Rutter, M. (1982) *Maternal Deprivation Re-assessed.* Penguin, Harmondsworth.
3. Bowlby, J. (1952) *Maternal Care and Mental Health*, 2nd ed. World Health Organization, Geneva.
4. Bowlby, J. (1953) *Child Care and the Growth of Love.* Pelican, Harmondsworth.
5. Robertson, J. (1970) *Young Children in Hospital.* Tavistock, London.
6. Butler, N.R. & Golding, J. (1986) *From Birth to Five.* Pergamon, Oxford.
7. Douglas, J. (1993) *Psychology and Nursing Children.* Macmillan, London.
8. Muller, D.J., Harris, P.J., Wattley, L. & Taylor, J.D. (1992) *Nursing Children: Psychology, research and practice*, 2nd ed. Chapman & Hall, London.
9. Ministry of Health (1959) *The Welfare of Children in Hospital* (Platt Report). HMSO, London.
10. Report of the Committee on Child Health Services (1976) *Fit For The Future* (Court Report). HMSO, London.

11. Department of Health (1991) *Welfare of Children and Young People in Hospital.* HMSO, London.
12. Sainsbury, C.P.Q., Gray, O.P., Cleary, J., Davies, M.M. & Rowlandson, P.H. (1986) Care by parents of their children in hospital. *Archives of Disease in Childhood*, **61**, 612–15.
13. Cleary, J., Gray, O.P., Hall, D., Rowlandson, P.H., Sainsbury, C.P.Q. & Davies, M.M. (1986) Parental involvement in the lives of children in hospital. *Archives of Disease in Childhood*, **61**, 779–87.
14. Belson, P. (1981) Alternatives to hospital care. *Nursing*, **23**, 1015–16.
15. Fletcher, B. (1981) Psychological upset in post-hospitalised children: A review of the literature. *Maternal Child Nursing Journal*, **10**, 185–95.
16. Adams, J., Gill, S. & McDonald, M. (1991) Reducing fear in hospital. *Nursing Times*, **87** (1), 62–4.
17. Jay, S.M., Elliott, C.H. & Ozolins, M. (1985) Behavioural management of children's distress during painful medical procedures. *Behavioural Research Therapy*, **23** (5), 513–20.
18. Ross, D. & Ross, S. (1988) *Childhood Pain: Current Issues, Research and Management.* Urban & Schwarzenburg, Baltimore.
19. Day, A. (1987) Can Mummy Come Too? *Nursing Times*, **83** (51), 51–2.
20. Coulson, D. (1987) *A Study of Parental Presence in the Anaesthetic Room During Paediatric Induction of Anaesthesia: The Parent and Child's View.* Unpublished undergraduate dissertation, Institute of Nursing Studies, University of Hull.
21. Hawthorne, P.J. (1974) *Nurse – I Want My Mummy.* Royal College of Nursing, London.
22. Evans, M. (1992) Extending the Parental Role. *Professional Nurse*, **7** (12), 774–6.
23. Jennings, K. (1986) Helping them face tomorrow. *Nursing Times*, **82**, 32–5.
24. Taylor, M.R.H. & O'Connor, P. (1989) Resident parents and shorter hospital stay. *Archives of Disease in Psychology*, **64**, 274–6.
25. Edwardson, S.R. (1983) The choice between hospital and home care for terminally ill children. *Nursing Research*, **32**, 29–34.
26. Steele, N.F. & Harrison, B. (1986) Technology assisted children: assessing discharge preparation. *Journal of Pediatric Nursing*, **1** (3), 150–58.
27. Andrews, M.M. & Nielson, D.W. (1988) Technology dependent children in the home. *Pediatric Nursing*, **14** (2), 111–14.
28. Vermillion, B.D., Ballentine, T.V.N. & Grosfield, J.L. (1979) The effective use of the parent care unit for infants on the surgical service. *Journal of Pediatric Surgery*, **14**, 321–4.
29. Campbell, M. (1987) Children with on-going health needs. *Nursing*, Third Series, **23**, 871–5.
30. Vass Fore, C. & Holmes,S.S. (1983) A care by parent unit revisited. *American Journal of Maternal/Child Nursing*, **8**, 408–10.
31. Casey, A. (1988) Partnership in practice. *Nursing Times*, **84** (44), 67–8.
32. Casey, A. (1988) Partnership with child and family. *Senior Nurse*, **8** (4), 8–9.
33. Bishop, J. (1988) Sharing the caring. *Nursing Times*, **84** (30), 60–61.
34. Dearmun, A. (1992) Perceptions of parental participation. *Paediatric Nursing*, **4** (7), 6–9.
35. Jolly, J. (1981) *The Other Side of Paediatrics.* Macmillan, London.
36. Fradd, E. (1988) Achieving new roles. *Nursing Times*, **84** (50), 38–40.
37. Glasper, A. (1990) Emancipation of parents. *Nursing Standard*, **4** (22), 25.

38. Gulseth Schepp, K. (1992) Correlates of mothers who prefer control over their hospitalised children's care. *Journal of Pediatric Nursing*, **7** (2), 83–9.

39. Knafi, I., Cavallarrii, K. & Dixon, D. (1988) *Paediatric Hospitalisation – Family and Nurse Perspectives*. Scott, Foresman & Co., London.

40. Webb, N., Hull, D. & Madely, R. (1985) Care by parents in hospital. *British Medical Journal*, **291**, 176–7.

41. Marriott, S. (1990) Parent Power. *Nursing Times*, **86** (34), 68.

42. Fradd, E. (1988) Achieving change in the clinical area: supporting innovation. *Senior Nurse*, **8** (12), 19–21.

43. Gill, K. (1987) Parent participation with a family health focus: Nurses' attitudes. *Paediatric Nursing*, **13** (2), 94–6.

44. Fradd, E. (1986) It's child's play. *Nursing Times*, **82** (41), 40–42.

Chapter 5
Nursing Action

The child's primary or named nurse prescribes nursing action or intervention that will lead to:

- an improvement or alleviation of the problem;
- helping the child and family meet their need(s).

The child and family's involvement in and contribution to the planning process is extremely important. The plan of care that is written in the 'Nursing Action' column (see Fig. 4.1) is discussed with the child and family in order to ensure that they fully understand the care that has been planned and why.

Negotiated care

The concept of negotiated care is seen as one of the vital components within the caring process. This is reflected in the nursing records (see Fig. 4.1). Once the plan of care has been written, the primary or named nurse negotiates the degree of participation that the child, parents and family wish to undertake with support and guidance from the nurse. The need to be flexible is recognized, as their participation will be affected by when they are able to visit, for example. However, specific measures and time frequencies concerning their agreed level of involvement must be recorded in the 'Child/Parent Action' column (see Fig. 4.1).

It should be noted that there is no obligation for the parents or the family to participate in care delivery and that they are able to opt in or out of care provision as they wish. For this reason care *must* be re-negotiated each day, with the action to be taken by the nurse or parent/carer stated clearly in the appropriate area of the Nursing Care Plan.

The child and parents (as appropriate) are asked to sign the Care Plan in the nurse/parent signature column to document that they agree with the information that has been recorded. The signatures *do not* indicate that the parents are taking responsibility for their child's care but that the Care Plan is a true record of the negotiated plan of care. It should be noted that some parents may choose not to sign the Care Plan.

As this is a legal document, it is imperative that the date and time of the plan of care is documented accurately and signed appropriately. Other members of the health care team, i.e. the dietician or physiotherapist, may include care that they have planned. They must, however, sign indicating their role and profession.

'Amend Action' column

The time, date and signature(s) must be recorded in the 'Amend Action' column (see Fig. 4.1) to document that 'one-off' care has been delivered or that care has been discontinued. The 'Amend Action' column is applicable to both the 'Nursing' and 'Child/Parent' column. When care has been discontinued in either column it must be crossed through, dated, timed and signed in the 'Amend Action' column.

Discharge planning guidelines

Preparation for discharge is extremely important. Good organization and communication may alleviate child and parental anxiety and ensure that discharge is not delayed unnecessarily. As many children remain in hospital for a short period of time this process needs to be considered as soon as possible. Discharge planning should, therefore, be considered on the day of admission. Or discharge planning may begin prior to admission, an example of which is when planned day case surgery patients receive post-operative information sheets with the admission letter.

The primary or named nurse co-ordinates the child and family's care, including potential discharge. Discharge planning ensures any potential problems such as transport difficulties are eliminated. Early referral to the community nursing team (if appropriate) will enable the team to develop relationships with the child and family whilst they are still in hospital and ensure that arrangements for equipment and home care are completed. Parent-held records and the discharge checklist on the child's history Sheet 2 (see Fig. 3.2) must be completed and signed by the nurse discharging the child and family.

The Problem Page Index

The Problem Page Index (Fig. 5.1) enables the rapid identification of a particular problem or Care Plan Sheet when the child has many problems or needs. It is an index of page numbers not a means of numbering problems, and as it is not an integral part of the nursing process records it is only used when appropriate. If it is used, it must be kept up-to-date and placed at the front of the nursing notes.

Fig. 5.1 The Problem Page Index.

PROBLEM PAGE INDEX

Please use one space only for one problem

Problem Sheet Number	Problem	Problem Outcome eg, Resolved	Date
1			
2			
3			
4			
5			
30			

Case study 2
Clare Brown: Planning for discharge on the day of admission

The following case study demonstrates the application of the Nottingham model, highlighting a child and family focused approach and the concept of negotiated care. In particular, this case study also demonstrates the use of the 'Amend Action' column and the value of early discharge planning.

Clare Brown, a 10-week-old baby, was admitted to Victoria Ward following a cyanotic and possible apnoeic episode. She was accompanied by her parents June and Tony Brown. Staff nurse Tina Dixon greeted them on arrival at the ward. Tina was to be Clare's primary nurse.

The completed History Sheet(s) (Figs 5.2 and 5.3) and the Communication Sheet (Fig. 5.4) indicate:

- That Clare's parents wish to be involved in her care.
- A lack of close friends and family support (the family has recently moved to Nottingham from Gloucester).
- Other factors within the family background, including June and Tony's infertility problems, two previous miscarriages and the fact that Clare was conceived by in vitro fertilization.

	CHILD'S HISTORY SHEET 1	
WARD: VICTORIA		REG NO: 748392
Family Name: BROWN	Date: 12/2/94 Time: 10.00	Family's perception of previous admission:
First Name: CLARE	Reason for admission:	HAS NOT BEEN IN HOSPITAL
Likes to be called: CLARE	LOSS OF COLOUR WHILST BEING FED	SINCE BIRTH
Age: 10/52		
DOB: 28-11-93	Accompanied by: MOTHER & FATHER	
Birth weight: 6lb 2oz	Why do the parents think the child has been admitted:	
Religion: C/E	WENT BLUE WHILST FEEDING ? STOPPED BREATHING	Parent(s) Carer(s) Resident: (YES)/NO
Child's Address: 19 TEWKESBURY CRESENT BRAMCOTE NOTTINGHAM		IN CUBICLE Where: (FAMILY CARE ASSISTANT ARRANGING DOUBLE Z BED)
Postcode: NG9 3FB	Medical Diagnosis: CYANOTIC EPISODE ? APNOEA	Likes to be known as: TONY & JUNE
		Do they wish to participate in the care of the child: YES - NORMAL BABY CARE & WOULD LIKE TO LEARN ANY ADDITIONAL PROCEDURES/CARE
Telephone No: 624689		
Next of Kin: TONY & JUNE BROWN	What reason does the child give for this admission:	
Relationship to child: PARENTS Address if different from above:		Social Arrangements: FATHER HAS ARRANGED TO HAVE TIME OFF WORK TO BE RESIDENT. RECENTLY MOVED TO AREA FROM GLOUCESTER - NO REAL FRIENDS IN NOTTINGHAM. MATERNAL GRANDMOTHER DUE TO VISIT & HAD PLANNED TO STAY FOR 2/52 NEXT DOOR NEIGHBOUR WILL FEED & EXERCISE 'RUPERT' - THE FAMILY DOG
AS ABOVE	TOO YOUNG	
Telephone No: Work: 268349 DAD Home: 624689	Previous relevant history/admissions: NO PREVIOUS MEDICAL PROBLEMS OR ADMISSIONS TO HOSPITAL	
With whom does the child reside: TONY & JUNE BROWN	BORN AT GREENWOLD GENERAL HOSPITAL, GLOUCESTER.	
Relationship to Child: PARENTS	FULL TERM NORMAL DELIVERY	Name and age of siblings:
Who has parental responsibility for this child?: MOTHER & FATHER		NO OTHER SIBLINGS
Telephone number: 624689		
Child's Nurse/Team: TINA DIXON	Consultant: DR BARD	

Fig. 5.2 Case study 2: History Sheet 1.

CHILD'S HISTORY SHEET 2

GP DR RODGERS Address HEALTH CENTRE, BRAMCOTE LANE, BRAMCOTE Tel No. 665510	Immunisation — Date or age administered: Dip] Tet] Polio Pert] — 1st 28/1/94; 2nd ....; 3rd	Referrals made whilst in hospital, contact — Sign / Date CAROL GREEN (CHILDREN'S UNIT HEALTH VISITOR) — T. DIXON 12/2/94 TOM STEWART (CHAPLAIN) — T. DIXON 12/2/94
Health Visitor RITA HAWLEY Address AS ABOVE Tel No. 665510	Measles/Mumps/Rubella ~~YES~~/NO Meningitis ~~YES~~/NO Booster Dip. Tet. Polio (pre-school) ~~YES~~/NO BCG Age administered	Checklist for discharge info & referrals
Health Centre Address BRAMCOTE LANE, BRAMCOTE Tel No. 665510	Booster Tet. & Polio School Leavers ~~YES~~/NO Date of last Tetanus AS PER TRIPLE Reason immunisations not given:	Sign / Date Parent/child informed — T. DIXON 13/2/94 Discharge advice sheet given — T. DIXON 12/2/94 Equipment loaned: APNOEA ALARM — T. DIXON 14/2/94
Social Worker/other contacts —		Ward appt given to family OPD appt given to family DR BARD 26/2/94 09.00 — T. DIXON 14/2/94
Other information PARENTS VERY ANXIOUS BOTH IN MID THIRTIES. HAD INVESTIGATIONS FOR INFERTILITY. CLARE CONCEIVED BY IVF. JUNE MISCARRIED TWO PREVIOUS PREGNANCIES	Recent Contact with infectious diseases NONE KNOWN	Health Visitor informed — T. DIXON 13/2/94 Community Nurse informed Social Worker
	Allergies NONE KNOWN	Doctor's Letter — T. DIXON 14/2/94
Ward Facilities - Tick box when explained to parents Parents' Kitchen ✓ Parents' Sitting/Smoking Room ✓ Ward Kitchen ✓ Parent information board/file ✓ Parent shower/toilet facilities ✓ Telephone ✓ Dining Room facilities ✓ Family Care Assistant ✓ Chaplaincy Department ✓ Fire Regulations ✓ Facilities re-explained on ward transfer	Current medications & method of administration NOT ON ANY MEDICATION HAS NEVER HAD ANY MEDICATION Signature of nurse taking history: T. DIXON — Date: 12/2/94 Signature of nurse checking: — Date:	Parent held records completed: Yes ✓ T. DIXON 14/2/94; No; N/A Discharge weight 3.6kg — T. DIXON 14/2/94 Medications Discharge Date 14/2/94 Time 11-00

Fig. 5.3 Case study 2: History Sheet 2.

CHILDREN'S UNIT NOTTINGHAM
COMMUNICATION SHEET

Child's Name CLARE BROWN .... Hospital No 748392

TIME	DATE	COMMUNICATION	SIGNATURE
10.30	12/2/94	EMERGENCY ADMISSION VIA CHILDREN'S ACCIDENT & EMERGENCY. LOSS OF COLOUR	
		WHILST FEEDING ? STOPPED BREATHING. PARENTS EXTREMELY ANXIOUS &	
		DISTRESSED. JUNE HAS HAD TWO PREVIOUS MISCARRIAGES. CLARE CONCEIVED	
		BY IVF.	T. DIXON
14.00	12/2/94	MATERNAL GRANDMOTHER TELEPHONED. WILL BE TRAVELLING TO NOTTINGHAM	
		TOMORROW.	T. DIXON

Fig. 5.4 Case study 2: Communication Sheet.

Fig. 5.5 (facing page) **Case study 2: Assessment Sheet (Gingerbread Man).**

The above factors have been highlighted as it is likely that they will not only affect June and Tony's ability to cope with Clare's admission and the development/adaptation of coping strategies, but also influence discharge planning. It is from the completed History Sheet(s) and the 'On Admission' section of the Gingerbread Man Assessment Sheet (Fig. 5.5) that the needs of Clare and her parents can be clearly identified.

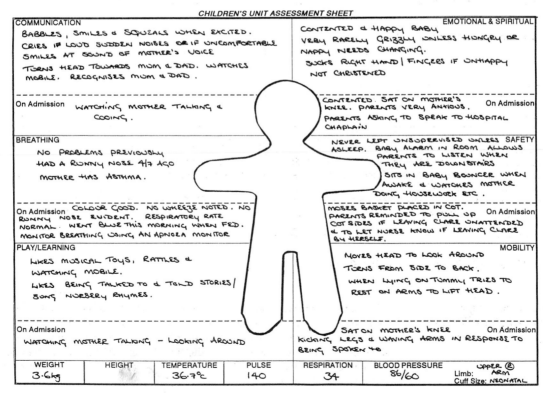

CHILDREN'S UNIT – ASSESSMENT SHEET

Name CLARE BROWN	Hosp No 748392	Date 12/2/94	Sign of Nurse Taking	Sign of Nurse Checking:
		Time 10.15	History: T. DIXON	

SLEEP AND COMFORT
SLEEPS IN MOSES BASKET IN SAME ROOM AS PARENTS.
COVERED WITH SMALL BLANKET & DUVET. SLEEPS ON
BACK.
DURING DAY - AWAKE FOR SHORT PERIODS BETWEEN
FEEDS. SMALL WHITE FURRY TEDDY TO HOLD.
LISTENS TO MUSICAL RADIO PRIOR TO SLEEPING

On Admission (Use Pain Scale if appropriate)
GRIZZLY LAST NIGHT - DIFFICULT TO
SETTLE. CONTENTED ON ADMISSION.

CONTROL OF BODY TEMPERATURE
HANDS & FEET SOMETIMES FEEL COLD.
WEARS MITS & HAT WHEN GOING OUT

On Admission
NORMAL BODY TEMPERATURE TO TOUCH.

WASHING/CARE OF SKIN/DRESSING
BATHED AT NIGHT - PARENTS TAKE IT IN TURNS TO
BATH. ENJOYS BATH - GETS EXCITED WHEN HEARS
RUNNING WATER. LIKES HAIR BEING WASHED.
'TOP & TAILED' IN THE MORNING & AS NECESSARY.
USES INFACARE. WEARS MOSTLY COTTON CLOTHES
AS TENDS TO DEVELOP A RASH OTHERWISE

On Admission HAD BATH LAST NIGHT
'TOP & TAILED' PRIOR TO FEED AT 08.30 THIS MORNING.
NO RASH / ECZEMA EVIDENT.
WILL WEAR OWN CLOTHES. PARENTS ADVISED RE:
WASHING FACILITIES.

EATING AND DRINKING
BREAST FED ON DEMAND
LAST WEEK STARTED HAVING SOME
BABY RICE MID- MORNING -
BUT DISLIKES IT.
WILL FEED FROM BOTTLE.

On Admission
LAST BREAST FED AT
08.30.
MOTHER WILL CONTINUE TO BREAST
FEED ON DEMAND & EXPRESS
BREAST MILK IF LEAVING THE WARD
FOR A PERIOD OF TIME.

ELIMINATION
WET NAPPIES X7 /DAY
BOX 3-4 /DAY - SOFT YELLOW STOOL
WEARS MINI DISPOSABLE NAPPIES
CRIES WHEN NAPPY NEEDS CHANGING

URINALYSIS
PH 7. NAD

On Admission
LAST WET NAPPY AT ABOUT 8AM
12/2/94. B.N.O. TODAY.
PARENTS HAVE BROUGHT OWN SUPPLY OF
DISPOSABLE NAPPIES

CHILDREN'S UNIT ASSESSMENT SHEET

COMMUNICATION
BABBLES, SMILES & SQUEALS WHEN EXCITED.
CRIES IF LOUD SUDDEN NOISES OR IF UNCOMFORTABLE
SMILES AT SOUND OF MOTHER'S VOICE
TURNS HEAD TOWARDS MUM & DAD. WATCHES
MOBILE. RECOGNISES MUM & DAD.

On Admission WATCHING MOTHER TALKING &
COOING.

BREATHING
NO PROBLEMS PREVIOUSLY
HAD A RUNNY NOSE 4/7 AGO
MOTHER HAS ASTHMA.

On Admission COLOUR GOOD. NO WHEEZE NOTED. NO
RUNNY NOSE EVIDENT. RESPIRATORY RATE
NORMAL. WENT BLUE THIS MORNING WHEN FED.
MONITOR BREATHING USING AN APNOEA MONITOR

PLAY/LEARNING
LIKES MUSICAL TOYS, RATTLES &
WATCHING MOBILE.
LIKES BEING TALKED TO & TOLD STORIES/
SONG NURSERY RHYMES.

On Admission
WATCHING MOTHER TALKING - LOOKING AROUND

EMOTIONAL & SPIRITUAL
CONTENTED & HAPPY BABY
VERY RARELY GRIZZLY UNLESS HUNGRY OR
NAPPY NEEDS CHANGING.
SUCKS RIGHT HAND / FINGERS IF UNHAPPY
NOT CHRISTENED

On Admission
CONTENTED. SAT ON MOTHER'S
KNEE. PARENTS VERY ANXIOUS.
PARENTS ASKING TO SPEAK TO HOSPITAL
CHAPLAIN

SAFETY
NEVER LEFT UNSUPERVISED UNLESS
ASLEEP. BABY ALARM IN ROOM ALLOWS
PARENTS TO LISTEN WHEN
THEY ARE DOWNSTAIRS
SITS IN BABY BOUNCER WHEN
AWAKE & WATCHES MOTHER
DOING HOUSEWORK ETC.

On Admission
MOSES BASKET PLACED IN COT.
PARENTS REMINDED TO PULL UP
COT SIDES IF LEAVING CLARE UNATTENDED
& TO LET NURSE KNOW IF LEAVING CLARE
BY HERSELF.

MOBILITY
MOVES HEAD TO LOOK AROUND
TURNS FROM SIDE TO BACK.
WHEN LYING ON TUMMY TRIES TO
REST ON ARMS TO LIFT HEAD.

On Admission
SAT ON MOTHER'S KNEE
KICKING LEGS & WAVING ARMS IN RESPONSE TO
BEING SPOKEN TO

WEIGHT	HEIGHT	TEMPERATURE	PULSE	RESPIRATION	BLOOD PRESSURE	UPPER (L) ARM
3.6kg		36.7°C	140	34	86/60	Limb:
						Cuff Size: NEONATAL

Fig. 5.6 (bottom and facing page) Case study 2: Nursing Care plan – breathing.

It can be seen that Clare's breathing will need to be monitored (Figs 5.6 and 5.7). In addition to the recording of four-hourly observations of Clare's respiratory rate, an apnoea monitor is to be used to assist in this purpose. June and Tony have expressed a desire to learn to record Clare's observations, and Tina has incorporated this into the plan of care. It should be noted that the plan of care emphasizes supporting and teaching June and Tony from the very outset. In particular, the plan centres around the use and functioning of the apnoea monitor in preparation for discharge. A Parent Information leaflet (see Appendix 1) is used as a means to reinforce the information given and to structure discharge planning. As each component is completed or arranged, Tina records this fact in the 'Amend Action' column, signing and entering the date and time that this has occurred. This then notifies others of the progress that has been achieved.

In view of the fact that Clare experienced difficulty in breathing whilst feeding, Tina has also formulated a plan of care that includes observing Clare while she is feeding (Figs 5.8 and 5.9). In addition, Tina recognizes the importance of reassuring June and encouraging her to continue breast-feeding Clare. The plan of care also includes contacting the health visitor for the Children's Unit and arranging for her to discuss weaning with June.

In recognition of Clare's parents' need for emotional support, Tina has written a plan of care to address their particular needs (Figs 5.10 and 5.11). The plan involves explaining procedures to them and providing them with opportunities to express their fears and discuss their feelings. Tina's plan includes contacting the health visitor for the Children's Unit who will then liaise with Clare's own health visitor in order to arrange for support upon her discharge. This undoubtedly

NURSING CARE PLAN

NAME: CLARE BROWN   HOSPITAL NO: 748392   AGE: 10/52

ACTIVITY OF LIVING: BREATHING   PROBLEM/NEED: LOSS OF COLOUR ? STOPPED BREATHING

DATE	TIME	NURSING ACTION	AMEND ACTION TIME, DATE AND SIGN	CHILD/PARENT ACTION	SIGN PARENT AND NURSE
12/2/94	10.30	* NURSE IN CUBICLE CLOSE TO THE NURSES STATION			
		* ENSURE OXYGEN & SUCTION ARE AVAILABLE & IN WORKING ORDER, NEAR CLARE'S COT	12/2/94 10.40 T. DIXON		
		* OBSERVE COLOUR OF LIPS & SKIN. REPORT TO MEDICAL STAFF IF CYANOSIS IS NOTED & TAKE APPROPRIATE ACTION AS REQUIRED			
		* OBSERVE CLARE FOR SIGNS OF CYANOSIS WHILST BEING FED			
		* RECORD 4 HOURLY OBSERVATIONS OF TEMPERATURE, PULSE &. RESPIRATIONS. NOTING & RECORDING THE RATE & DEPTH OF RESPIRATIONS. REPORT TO MEDICAL STAFF ANY ABNORMALITIES OR CHANGES IN CONDITION		JUNE & TONY WILL RECORD CLARE'S TEMPERATURE, PULSE & RESPIRATIONS FOLLOWING INSTRUCTION & UNDER SUPERVISION & WITH SUPPORT	T. BROWN J. BROWN
		* MONITOR RESPIRATION WITH THE USE OF AN APNOEA MONITOR. NOTE & RECORD APNOEIC EPISODES. REPORT TO MEDICAL STAFF & TAKE APPROPRIATE ACTION AS REQUIRED.			
					T. DIXON
				The signature of the parent indicates that this care plan has been negotiated	

NURSING CARE PLAN

NAME	CLARE BROWN		HOSPITAL NO.	748392		AGE	10/52

ACTIVITY OF LIVING	BREATHING		PROBLEM/NEED	LOSS OF COLOUR ? STOPPED BREATHING

DATE	TIME	NURSING ACTION	AMEND ACTION TIME, DATE AND SIGN	CHILD/PARENT ACTION	SIGN PARENT AND NURSE
12/2/94	10.30	* DISCUSS & EXPLAIN / PARENT INFORMATION LEAFLET RE: APNOEA ALARM WITH TONY & JUNE	T. DIXON 12/2/94 11.30		
		* DEMONSTRATE THE / SOUND OF THE ALARM & ENSURE / THAT TONY & JUNE FULLY UNDERSTAND HOW THE APNOEA ALARM OPERATES. DISCUSS THE / POSSIBLE REASONS WHY IT MAY ALARM & THE ACTION TO BE TAKEN	T. DIXON 12/2/94 11.30	TONY & JUNE AWARE THAT THEY CAN ASK FOR FURTHER DEMONSTRATIONS / EXPLANATIONS IF THEY WISH	T. BROWN J. BROWN
		* ARRANGE FOR MEDICAL / STAFF TO DISCUSS / DEMONSTRATE THE ACTION TO BE TAKEN IN THE EVENT OF AN APNOEIC ATTACK (AS PER PARENT INFORMATION LEAFLET)	12/2/94 13.00 T. DIXON		
		* SHOW TONY & JUNE / THE VIDEO 'THE BREATH OF LIFE' & ANSWER ANY QUESTIONS TONY & JUNE MAY HAVE	T. DIXON 13/2/94 15.00	TONY & JUNE TO VIEW THE VIDEO	T. BROWN J. BROWN
		* PROVIDE TONY & JUNE WITH THE APPROPRIATE SUPPLIES OF SENSORS & TAPE	13/2/94 20.00 T. DIXON		
		* WITH TONY & JUNE / COMPLETE AN INDEMNITY FORM FOR THE LOAN OF THE APNOEA ALARM	T. DIXON 14/2/94 10.00		
					T. DIXON

The signature of the parent indicates that this care plan has been negotiated

NURSING CARE PLAN

NAME	CLARE BROWN		HOSPITAL NO.	748392		AGE	10/52

ACTIVITY OF LIVING	BREATHING		PROBLEM/NEED	LOSS OF COLOUR ? STOPPED BREATHING

DATE	TIME	NURSING ACTION	AMEND ACTION TIME, DATE AND SIGN	CHILD/PARENT ACTION	SIGN PARENT AND NURSE
12/2/94	10.30	* RE-CHECK THAT TONY & JUNE FULLY UNDERSTAND THE CONTENT OF THE PARENT INFORMATION LEAFLET, OFFER FURTHER INSTRUCTION / AS REQUIRED.	T. DIXON 14/2/94 10.00	TONY & JUNE AWARE THAT THEY CAN ASK FOR FURTHER INSTRUCTION & ASK QUESTIONS	T. BROWN J. BROWN
		* ARRANGE OUT PATIENT APPOINTMENT & FOLLOW UP CARE AS APPROPRIATE	T. DIXON 13/2/94 16.00		T. DIXON

The signature of the parent indicates that this care plan has been negotiated

assists with Clare's early discharge from hospital. In addition, contact with Clare's maternal grandmother results in the grandmother making an earlier than planned visit to Nottingham, thereby ensuring that June and Tony will have adequate support and assistance upon Clare's discharge from hospital.

This particular case study highlights the benefit of planning for discharge on the day of admission and the use of a Parent Information Sheet to structure this process, thereby ensuring that parents receive the teaching and information to enable early discharge.

NURSING CARE PLAN – PROGRESS UPDATE

NAME CLARE BROWN   HOSPITAL NO 748 392   AGE 10/52

ACTIVITY OF LIVING BREATHING   PROBLEM/NEED LOSS OF COLOUR? STOPPED BREATHING

DATE	TIME		SIGN
12/2/94	10·15	COLOUR GOOD ON ADMISSION. BASELINE OBSERVATIONS WITHIN NORMAL LIMITS	T. DIXON
12/2/94	11·30	PARENT INFORMATION LEAFLET RE: APNOEA ALARM DISCUSSED WITH TONY & JUNE.	
		DEMONSTRATED HOW THE APNOEA ALARM OPERATES.	T. DIXON
12/2/94	13·00	DR WHITE CONTACTED. WILL DISCUSS & DEMONSTRATE THE ACTION TO BE TAKEN IN	
		THE EVENT OF AN APNOEIC ATTACK WITH TONY & JUNE TOMORROW AT 14·00.	
		TONY & JUNE INFORMED.	T. DIXON
12/2/94	14·00	COLOUR GOOD. NO CYANOSIS OBSERVED.	T. DIXON
12/2/94	21·00	OBSERVATIONS RECORDED AS CHARTED. STABLE & SATISFACTORY. NO APNOEIC	
		EPISODES NOTED	J. TODD
13/2/94	07·00	NO SIGNS OF CYANOSIS WHILST FEEDING. NO APNOEA'S. OBSERVATIONS STABLE	C. SMITH
13/2/94	12·30	OBSERVATIONS RECORDED. WITHIN NORMAL LIMITS. COLOUR REMAINS GOOD.	B. DOLAN
13/2/94	14·30	THE ACTION TO BE TAKEN IN THE EVENT OF AN APNOEIC ATTACK DISCUSSED WITH	
		TONY & JUNE BY DR WHITE	T. DIXON
13/2/94	15·00	TONY & JUNE SHOWN THE VIDEO 'THE BREATH OF LIFE'	T. DIXON
13/2/94	15·45	SEEN BY DR BAIRD. CAN BE DISCHARGED HOME TOMORROW IF NO APNOEIC	
		SPELLS & IF JUNE & TONY ARE HAPPY.	T. DIXON
13/2/94	16·00	OUTPATIENT APPOINTMENT ARRANGED FOR 26/2/94 @ 09·00. RITA HAWLEY	
		(CLARE'S HEALTH VISITOR) CONTACTED & INFORMED OF POTENTIAL DISCHARGE, WILL	
		VISIT CLARE AT HOME ON 15/2/94 AT SOME TIME DURING THE AFTERNOON.	
		TONY & JUNE INFORMED	T. DIXON
13/2/94	18·00	COLOUR REMAINS GOOD. OBSERVATIONS STABLE & SATISFACTORY	T. DIXON
13/2/94	20·00	TONY & JUNE GIVEN APPROPRIATE SUPPLIES FOR THE APNOEA MONITOR.	T. DIXON
14/2/94	06·50	NO CYANOTIC OR APNOEIC PERIODS. OBSERVATIONS WITHIN NORMAL LIMITS	C. SMITH
14/2/94	10·00	OBSERVATIONS STABLE & SATISFACTORY. SEEN BY DR WHITE. PARENTS HAPPY	
		TO TAKE CLARE HOME. INDEMNITY FORM COMPLETED. REVIEWED CONTENT OF	
		PARENT INFORMATION LEAFLET WITH TONY & JUNE. GIVEN OUT PATIENT	
		APPOINTMENT & GP LETTER	T. DIXON
14/2/94	11·00	DISCHARGED HOME	T. DIXON

Fig. 5.7 Case Study 2: Progress Update – breathing.

NURSING CARE PLAN

NAME	CLARE BROWN		HOSPITAL NO.	748392		AGE	10/52

ACTIVITY OF LIVING	EATING & DRINKING	PROBLEM/NEED	LOSS OF COLOUR WHILST BEING FED

DATE	TIME	NURSING ACTION	AMEND ACTION TIME, DATE AND SIGN	CHILD/PARENT ACTION	SIGN PARENT AND NURSE
12/2/94	10·30	* WEIGH ON ADMISSION & THEN TWICE A WEEK (TUES & FRI)			
		* SUPPORT JUNE TO CONTINUE BREAST FEEDING CLARE ON DEMAND			
		* RECORD BREAST FEEDS ON FLUID BALANCE CHART		JUNE TO RECORD ON FLUID BALANCE CHART WHEN CLARE HAS BEEN BREAST FED	J. BROWN
		* OBSERVE WHILST FEEDING, NOTING & REPORTING IF CLARE HAS ANY DIFFICULTIES FEEDING			
		* SHOW JUNE THE FACILITIES AVAILABLE TO EXPRESS BREAST MILK & HOW & WHERE THIS CAN BE STORED - ENSURING THAT THIS HAS BEEN ACCURATELY LABELLED.	T. DIXON 12/2/94 11·00		
		* ENSURE THAT JUNE IS SHOWN THE FACILITIES ON THE WARD WHERE SHE CAN MAKE HERSELF DRINKS & THEREBY ENSURE A GOOD FLUID INTAKE	T. DIXON 12/2/94 11·00		
		* CONTACT THE CHILDREN'S UNIT HEALTH VISITOR & ARRANGE FOR HER TO DISCUSS WEANING WITH JUNE	T. DIXON 12/2/94 11·20		T. DIXON

The signature of the parent indicates that this care plan has been negotiated

Fig. 5.8 Case study 2: Nursing Care Plan – eating and drinking.

NURSING CARE PLAN – PROGRESS UPDATE

NAME	CLARE BROWN		HOSPITAL NO	748392		AGE	10/52

DATE	TIME	ACTIVITY OF LIVING	EATING & DRINKING	PROBLEM/NEED	LOSS OF COLOUR WHILST BEING FED	SIGN

DATE	TIME	(ACTIVITY OF LIVING EATING & DRINKING ... PROBLEM/NEED LOSS OF COLOUR WHILST BEING FED)	SIGN
12/2/94	11·00	JUNE SHOWN THE FACILITIES AVAILABLE TO EXPRESS BREAST MILK & THOSE AVAILABLE ON THE WARD FOR MAKING DRINKS	T. DIXON
12/2/94	11·20	CHILDREN'S UNIT HEALTH VISITOR CONTACTED. WILL VISIT WARD TO TALK TO JUNE RE: WEANING	T. DIXON
12/2/94	12·00	BREAST FED FOR 15-20 MINS. NO DIFFICULTIES NOTED	T. DIXON
12/2/94	17·00	CAROL GREEN VISITED. DISCUSSED WEANING WITH JUNE	J. TODD
12/2/94	21·00	FEEDING WELL. NO DIFFICULTIES EXPERIENCED WHILST BEING FED	J. TODD
13/2/94	07·00	FED ON DEMAND OVERNIGHT. NO DIFFICULTIES	C. SMITH
13/2/94	12·30	CONTINUES TO FEED WELL. NO DIFFICULTIES OBSERVED DURING FEEDING	B. DOLAN
13/2/94	21·00	BREAST FEEDING WELL.	T. DIXON
14/2/94	06·50	BREAST FED AS CHARTED ON FLUID BALANCE CHART. NO DIFFICULTIES NOTED	C. SMITH
14/2/94	10·00	FED WELL THIS MORNING. NO DIFFICULTIES OBSERVED	T. DIXON
14/2/94	11·00	DISCHARGED HOME	T. DIXON

Fig. 5.9 Case study 2: Progress Update – eating and drinking.

NURSING CARE PLAN

NAME CLARE BROWN	HOSPITAL NO. 748392	AGE 10/52

ACTIVITY OF LIVING EMOTIONAL / SPIRITUAL

PROBLEM/NEED CLARE ? STOPPED BREATHING & HER PARENTS REQUIRE EMOTIONAL SUPPORT IN ORDER TO CARE FOR HER

DATE	TIME	NURSING ACTION	AMEND ACTION TIME, DATE AND SIGN	CHILD/PARENT ACTION	SIGN PARENT AND NURSE
12/2/94	10.30	* INTRODUCE SELF & OTHER MEMBERS OF STAFF TO CLARE & HER FAMILY			
		* SHOW CLARE'S PARENTS AROUND THE WARD & THE FACILITIES AVAILABLE FOR THEM	T. DIXON 12/2/94 11.00		
		* CONTACT THE FAMILY CARE ASSISTANT TO ARRANGE A DOUBLE Z BED	T. DIXON 12/2/94 11.20		
		* ENCOURAGE & SUPPORT CLARE'S PARENTS TO BE INVOLVED IN HER CARE AS MUCH AS THEY WISH & FEEL ABLE TO.		JANE & TONY AGREE TO PARTICIPATE IN CLARE'S CARE AS MUCH AS POSSIBLE & WILL PERFORM HER 'NORMAL' CARE WHEN PRESENT	J. BROWN T. BROWN
		* KEEP CLARE'S PARENTS INFORMED OF HER CONDITION, TREATMENT & PROGRESS			
		* EXPLAIN ALL PROCEDURES & INVESTIGATIONS TO CLARE & HER PARENTS		JANE & TONY WILL ASK QUESTIONS OR ASK TO SPEAK TO A DOCTOR WHENEVER THEY WISH	
		* ALLOW, ENABLE & SUPPORT CLARE'S PARENTS TO EXPRESS THEIR FEELINGS & TO DISCUSS THEIR FEARS			J. BROWN T. BROWN
		* PROVIDE OPPORTUNITIES FOR CLARE'S PARENTS TO ASK QUESTIONS & ANSWER ANY QUERIES THEY HAVE. REFER TO THE NURSE IN CHARGE OR THE DOCTOR AS REQUIRED			T. DIXON

The signature of the parent indicates that this care plan has been negotiated

NURSING CARE PLAN

NAME CLARE BROWN	HOSPITAL NO. 748392	AGE 10/52

ACTIVITY OF LIVING EMOTIONAL / SPIRITUAL

PROBLEM/NEED CLARE ? STOPPED BREATHING & HER PARENTS REQUIRE EMOTIONAL SUPPORT IN ORDER TO CARE FOR HER

DATE	TIME	NURSING ACTION	AMEND ACTION TIME, DATE AND SIGN	CHILD/PARENT ACTION	SIGN PARENT AND NURSE
12/2/94	10.30	* CONTACT THE HOSPITAL CHAPLAIN FOR SPIRITUAL & EMOTIONAL SUPPORT	T. DIXON 12/2/94 11.20		
		* CONTACT THE CHILDREN'S UNIT HEALTH VISITOR & ARRANGE FOR HER TO MEET CLARE'S PARENTS	T. DIXON 12/2/94 11.20		
					T. DIXON

The signature of the parent indicates that this care plan has been negotiated

Fig. 5.10 Case study 2: Nursing Care Plan – emotional/spiritual.

NURSING CARE PLAN – PROGRESS UPDATE

DATE	TIME	ACTIVITY OF LIVING EMOTIONAL/SPIRITUAL PROBLEM/NEED CLARE'S PARENTS NEED EMOTIONAL SUPPORT	SIGN
		NAME ... CLARE BROWN ...... HOSPITAL NO ...748392... AGE 10/52	
12/2/94	11·00	CLARE'S PARENTS SHOWN AROUND THE WARD & FACILITIES AVAILABLE	T. DIXON
12/2/94	11·20	FAMILY CARE ASSISTANT CONTACTED TO ARRANGE DOUBLE Z BED. CHILDREN'S UNIT	
		HEALTH VISITOR CONTACTED. WILL VISIT WARD TO TALK TO CLARE'S PARENTS.	
		HOSPITAL CHAPLAIN CONTACTED. WILL VISIT ABOUT 12·30. JUNE & TONY INFORMED	T. DIXON
12/2/94	13·00	TOM STEWART (HOSPITAL CHAPLAIN) VISITED. WILL RETURN TOMORROW.	T. DIXON
12/2/94	17·00	CAROL GREEN VISITED. SPOKE TO JUNE & TONY. WILL LIAISE WITH CLARE'S HEALTH	
		VISITOR TO PROVIDE FOLLOW UP SUPPORT AT HOME	J. TODD
13/2/94	03·00	PARENTS EXTREMELY ANXIOUS. UNABLE TO SLEEP. REASSURED & FEARS ALLAYED	C. SMITH
13/2/94	12·00	TOM STEWART VISITED	B. DOLAN
13/2/94	17·00	MATERNAL GRANDMOTHER ARRIVED FROM GLOUCESTER. WILL BE STAYING AT THE	
		FAMILY HOME. PLANS TO STAY FOR 2/52 TO GIVE SUPPORT TO JUNE & TONY	T. DIXON
14/2/94	06·50	PARENTS LESS ANXIOUS. REASSURED BY PRESENCE OF APNOEA MONITOR	C. SMITH
14/2/94	10·00	PARENTS MORE RELAXED. MATERNAL GRANDMOTHER VISITING	T. DIXON
14/2/94	11·00	DISCHARGED HOME. WARD CONTACT TELEPHONE NUMBER GIVEN. ADVISED TO	
		RING IF CONCERNED OR IF THEY HAVE FURTHER QUERIES	T. DIXON

Fig. 5.11 Case study 2: Progress Update – emotional/spiritual.

Chapter 6
Review of Nursing Action and Assessment of Progress

Care provision should not only be relevant but also appropriately and carefully considered so as to meet the needs of the individual child and family. Therefore, reviewing care and its outcome is of paramount importance. The care planned and recorded in the 'Nursing' and 'Child/Parent Action' column(s) is reviewed and updated. Information regarding alterations or progress is recorded on the reverse of the Care Plan or on a continuation sheet of the Progress Update Sheet. The Progress Update Sheet (Fig. 6.1) is used to record factual and concise information regarding the implementation and continuation of care, as well as a review of the outcomes of the care provided for the child and family.

NURSING CARE PLAN – PROGRESS UPDATE

NAME		HOSPITAL NO		AGE	
DATE	TIME	ACTIVITY OF LIVING .... PROBLEM/NEED			SIGN

Fig. 6.1 Progress Update Sheet.

The primary, associate or named nurse responsible for the child must assess and review care regularly throughout the shift. If the primary nurse is not available to update the Care Plan, any alterations must be clearly recorded for his/her attention when next on duty. This review includes both the Care Plans and the child's usual Activities of Living from the Assessment Sheet. Information regarding the latter, e.g. bathing and feeding, is recorded on the infant feed chart and/or Communication Sheet as appropriate. A review of relevant care can also be undertaken by other members of the health care team following discussion with either the named nurse or primary nurse.

It is important that an entry on the Progress Update Sheet is made on all Care Plans during each shift so as to demonstrate that the care that was planned has been delivered. When an entry has been made, the date and time must be recorded and signed. Double-sided Progress Update Sheets enable the review of a particular problem to continue in chronological order. However, it should be noted that it is extremely important that the 'problem' is recorded at the top of this sheet.

Communication Sheet

A Communication Sheet (Fig. 6.2), although not necessary for every child, allows the nurse to record any extra information that does not pertain to a specific problem, e.g. dates and times of telephone calls from the family or enquiries from other agencies. The Communication Sheet can also be used to record a summary of the child's previous nursing or medical history if the space on the History Sheet (see Fig. 3.1) is insufficient.

		CHILDREN'S UNIT NOTTINGHAM COMMUNICATION SHEET	
Child's Name			Hospital No ....
TIME	DATE	COMMUNICATION	SIGNATURE

Fig. 6.2 Communication Sheet.

The communication process

Communication between colleagues is extremely important in the care planning and care delivery process, and includes verbal communication at handover(s) (Fig. 6.3) and written communication via the nursing records. Feelings may be communicated verbally at handover, but written communication must always be factual and concise.

Fig. 6.3 Bedside communication at handover.

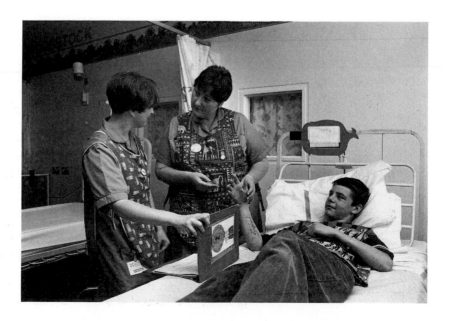

Case Study 3
Donna Jones: the importance of communication between professionals and parents

The following case study demonstrates the application of the Nottingham model to an Intensive Care situation and the importance of communication between health care professionals and with the child's family. It also highlights the adaptation of the Gingerbread Man Assessment Sheet for use within critical care areas.

Donna Jones, an 11-year-old, was admitted to the Children's Intensive Care Unit following a road traffic accident in which she sustained a severe closed head injury. Donna was transferred from Blankton General Hospital and accompanied by her parents Linda and Tony Jones.

The completed History Sheets (Figs 6.4 and 6.5) and the Communication Sheet (Fig. 6.6) indicate:

	CHILD'S HISTORY SHEET 1	
WARD: PICU		REG NO: 963148
Family Name: JONES	Date: 28|5|93 Time: 18 15	Family's perception of previous admission:
First Name: DONNA	Reason for admission:	PARENTS HAPPY WITH PREVIOUS ADMISSION & CARE AT THE LOCAL
Likes to be called: DONNA	DONNA RAN IN FRONT OF A CAR ON THE WAY HOME FROM SCHOOL	HOSPITAL.
Age: 11 YEARS		MOM STAYED AT DONNA'S BEDSIDE
DOB: 12·4·81	Accompanied by: PARENTS	& HELPED CARE FOR HER
Birth weight: 7lb 6oz	Why do the parents think the child has	
Religion: RIC	been admitted:	
Child's Address: 17 FIR AVENUE BOSTON LINCS	BECAUSE OF THE ACCIDENT, BAD INJURY TO HER HEAD	Parent(s) Carer(s) Resident: YES/NO
		Where: PARENTS UNIT - ROOM 4
Postcode: LE3 5AZ	Medical Diagnosis: MAJOR HEAD INJURY # BASE OF SKULL, BRUISES & LACERATIONS TO FACE & TRUNK	Likes to be known as: LINDA & TONY
		Do they wish to participate in the care of the child:
Telephone No: 75- 832791		YES, WOULD LIKE TO HELP
Next of Kin: LINDA & TONY JONES	What reason does the child give for	WASH HER
Relationship to child: PARENTS	this admission:	
Address if different from above:	NOT ABLE TO COMMUNICATE	Social Arrangements:
SAME ADDRESS	AS UNCONSCIOUS	OWN HOME, CENTRALLY HEATED.
		OWN TRANSPORT.
		MATERNAL GRANDPARENTS CARING
Telephone No:	Previous relevant history/admissions:	FOR SARAH AT THEIR HOME.
Work: 75-663472 DAD Home: AS ABOVE	MAY 1979- APPENDICECTOMY	
With whom does the child reside: LINDA, TONY & SARAH JONES		
Relationship to Child: PARENTS & SISTER		Name and age of siblings:
Who has parental responsibility for this child?: PARENTS		SARAH AGED 9YRS
Telephone number: AS ABOVE		
Child's Nurse/Team: CHRIS BROWN	Consultant: MR FRY	

Fig. 6.4 Case study 3: History Sheet 1.

CHILD'S HISTORY SHEET 2					
GP DR FREEMAN Address THE SURGERY PARK ROAD BOSTON, LINCS Tel No. 75-854361	Immunisation Dip] Tet] Polio Pert]	Date or age administered: 1st ✓ .... 2nd ✓ .... 3rd ✓	Referrals made whilst in hospital, contact TOM DREW (R/C PRIEST)	Sign C.BROWN	Date 28/5/93
Health Visitor Address N/A	Measles/Mumps/Rubella Meningitis Booster Dip. Tet. Polio (pre-school)	YES/NO YES/NO YES/NO			
Tel No.	BCG Age administered	MAY '79	Checklist for discharge info & referrals		
Health Centre Address GP SURGERY AS ABOVE	Booster Tet. & Polio School Leavers Date of last Tetanus	YES/NO MAY '79		Sign	Date
			Parent/child informed Discharge advice sheet given Equipment loaned		
Tel No.	Reason immunisations not given:				
Social Worker/other contacts			Ward appt given to family OPD appt given to family		
Other information TONY'S FATHER HAD A HEART ATTACK ONE MONTH AGO, NOW RECOVERING AT HOME	Recent Contact with infectious diseases NONE KNOWN		Health Visitor informed Community Nurse informed Social Worker		
	Allergies NONE KNOWN		Doctor's Letter		
Ward Facilities - Tick box when explained to parents	Current medications & method of administration		Parent held records completed:		
Parents' Kitchen ✓	NONE			Yes	
Parents' Sitting/Smoking Room ✓	DONNA IS UNABLE TO SWALLOW TABLETS			No	
Ward Kitchen ✓				N/A	
Parent information board/file ✓			Discharge weight		
Parent shower/toilet facilities ✓			Medications		
Telephone ✓					
Dining Room facilities ✓					
Family Care Assistant TO BE CONTACTED 29/5/93	Signature of nurse taking history: C. BROWN	Date: 28/5/93			
Chaplaincy Department ✓					
Fire Regulations ✓	Signature of nurse checking:	Date:			
Facilities re-explained on ward transfer			Discharge Date	Time	

Fig. 6.5 Case study 3: History Sheet 2.

CHILDREN'S UNIT NOTTINGHAM
COMMUNICATION SHEET

Child's Name DONNA JONES   Hospital No 963148

TIME	DATE	COMMUNICATION	SIGNATURE
20.50	28/5/93	TRANSFER FROM BLANKTON GENERAL HOSPITAL FOLLOWING RTA, SUSTAINING MAJOR	
		HEAD INJURY & NUMEROUS LACERATIONS TO TRUNK	
		ON ADMISSION: INTUBATED & SEDATED. IV INFUSION OF PLASMA IN PROGRESS	
		SEEN BY MR FRY - TO FOLLOW THE HEAD INJURY PROTOCOL	
		ATRACURIUM INFUSION COMMENCED & NURSED ON COOLING MATTRESS.	
		PARENTS SPOKEN TO BY MR FRY, SEVERITY OF INJURY, PROPOSED CARE & THE	
		POSSIBILITY THAT DONNA MAY NOT SURVIVE EXPLAINED TO THEM	
		P.C WILLIAMS ENQUIRED BY PHONE RE: DONNA'S CONDITION. PHONE CALL	
		RETURNED. STATEMENT GIVEN - IN AGREEMENT WITH PARENTS - AS 'CRITICALLY	
		ILL'. INFORMATION RECORDED IN THE POLICE BOOK.	C. BROWN
21.15	28/5/93	PRESS STATEMENT GIVEN: 'CRITICALLY ILL' AS DISCUSSED & AGREED WITH	
		DONNA'S PARENTS	C. BROWN

Fig. 6.6 Case study 3: Communication Sheet.

Fig. 6.7 (facing page)
Case study 3: Critical
Care Assessment Sheet.

- The parents' understanding of a life-threatening situation.
- That Donna and her parents have been exposed to a previous hospital admission.
- That Donna's parents wish to be involved in her care.
- The extent of the family's support network and arrangements for Sarah's (Donna's sister) care.
- Other stressful events in the family's life, i.e. paternal grandfather's heart attack.

These factors have been highlighted as they will undoubtedly affect the family's ability to cope with the situation, and the development/adaptation of coping strategies.

The Gingerbread Man Assessment Sheet (Fig. 6.7) has been specifically adapted for critical care areas. As the time taken for the admission procedure in the Children's Intensive Care Unit varies considerably and may cross over shifts, the Assessment Sheet becomes a communication sheet. It may be ticked or circled to facilitate completion. Detailed information is expected to be added when the initial urgency has passed and before the admitting nurse goes off-duty. It should be noted that although the boxes relating to Donna's normal Activities of Living remain empty at this point, as indicated in the guidelines (see chapter 3), these must be completed within 24 hours of Donna's admission. However, it is from the 'On Admission' section of the Gingerbread Man Assessment Sheet that Donna's needs can be clearly identified. It can be seen that Donna will require invasive monitoring and full nursing care, the priority being artificial ventilation in order to maintain respiration and oxygenation. The plan of care (Figs 6.8 and 6.9) demonstrates that this involves:

- The maintenance of a patent airway via an endotracheal tube using hourly suction.
- Correct positioning of the tube and ensuring the endotracheal tube is secure.
- Observing the chest movement for equal air entry.
- Monitoring oxygenation via an oxygen saturation monitor and blood gas analysis via the arterial line.
- Accurate recording of the ventilator settings hourly and liaising with the anaesthetist.

Whilst Donna requires invasive monitoring her safety needs are of paramount importance. These needs must be individually identified and the action/nursing observation required for each of these accurately documented within the plan of care, as in the case of the arterial line (Figs 6.10 and 6.11).

In relation to the Activities of Living, other requirements can be identified, including those related to eating and drinking. Figures 6.12 and 6.13 highlight the plan of care devised by Chris Brown (Donna's named nurse) in respect of maintaining hydration via the administration of intravenous fluids.

Admission to a critical care area is extremely stressful for the child's parents and family. In order to assist the family to come to terms with the current situation and develop coping strategies, they need to be supported, involved in Donna's care and kept informed of all changes in her care/treatment and condition, whilst also allowing them to express their fears and anxieties. The plan of care depicted in Figs 6.14 and 6.15 addresses the family's need for emotional and spiritual support, as well as Donna's need for reassurance and stimulation. As indicated by the History Sheet 1 (Fig. 6.4) and the plan of care, Donna's

CHILDREN'S UNIT – CRITICAL CARE AREAS ASSESSMENT SHEET

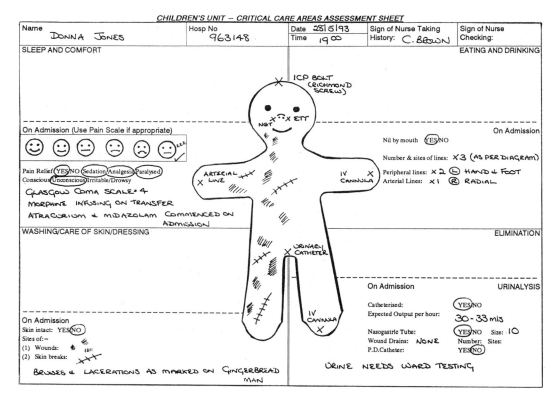

| Name DONNA JONES | Hosp No 963148 | Date 28|5|93 Time 1900 | Sign of Nurse Taking History: C. BROWN | Sign of Nurse Checking: |

SLEEP AND COMFORT / **EATING AND DRINKING**

ICP BOLT (RICHMOND SCREW)

NGT — ETT

On Admission (Use Pain Scale if appropriate)

😊 🙂 😐 🙁 😣 😫 ᶻᶻ ✓

Pain Relief YES/NO (Sedation) (Analgesia) (Paralysed)
Conscious (Unconscious) Irritable/Drowsy
GLASGOW COMA SCALE: 4
MORPHINE INFUSING ON TRANSFER
ATRACURIUM & MIDAZOLAM COMMENCED ON ADMISSION

EATING AND DRINKING

On Admission

Nil by mouth (YES)/NO

Number & sites of lines: X3 (AS PER DIAGRAM)

ARTERIAL LINE

IV CANNULA

Peripheral lines: X2 (L) HAND & FOOT
Arterial Lines: X1 (R) RADIAL

WASHING/CARE OF SKIN/DRESSING / **ELIMINATION**

URINARY CATHETER

IV CANNULA

On Admission
Skin intact: YES/(NO)
Sites of:–
(1) Wounds:
(2) Skin breaks:
BRUISES & LACERATIONS AS MARKED ON GINGERBREAD MAN

ELIMINATION

On Admission — URINALYSIS

Catheterised: (YES)/NO
Expected Output per hour: 30 – 33 mls

Nasogastric Tube: (YES)/NO Size: 10
Wound Drains: NONE Number: Sites:
P.D.Catheter: YES/(NO)

URINE NEEDS WARD TESTING

CHILDREN'S UNIT – CRITICAL CARE ASSESSMENT SHEET

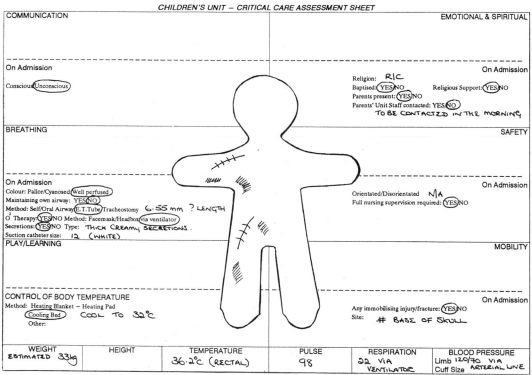

COMMUNICATION / **EMOTIONAL & SPIRITUAL**

On Admission

Conscious (Unconscious)

EMOTIONAL & SPIRITUAL

On Admission

Religion: R/C
Baptised: (YES)/NO   Religious Support: (YES)/NO
Parents present: (YES)/NO
Parents' Unit Staff contacted: YES/(NO)
TO BE CONTACTED IN THE MORNING

BREATHING / **SAFETY**

On Admission
Colour: Pallor/Cyanosed/(Well perfused)
Maintaining own airway: YES/(NO)
Method: Self/Oral Airway/(E.T.Tube)/Tracheostomy 6.55 mm ? LENGTH
O₂ Therapy: (YES)/NO Method: Facemask/Headbox/(via ventilator)
Secretions: (YES)/NO Type: THICK CREAMY SECRETIONS.
Suction catheter size: 12 (WHITE)

SAFETY

On Admission

Orientated/Disorientated N/A
Full nursing supervision required: (YES)/NO

PLAY/LEARNING / **MOBILITY**

CONTROL OF BODY TEMPERATURE
Method: Heating Blanket – Heating Pad
(Cooling Bed) COOL TO 32°C
Other:

MOBILITY

On Admission

Any immobilising injury/fracture: (YES)/NO
Site: # BASE OF SKULL

| WEIGHT ESTIMATED 33kg | HEIGHT | TEMPERATURE 36.2°C (RECTAL) | PULSE 98 | RESPIRATION 22 VIA VENTILATOR | BLOOD PRESSURE Limb 120/70 VIA ARTERIAL LINE Cuff Size |

NURSING CARE PLAN

NAME	DONNA JONES		HOSPITAL NO.	963 148		AGE 11 YEARS

ACTIVITY OF LIVING ... SAFETY

PROBLEM/NEED ... DONNA HAS A HEAD INJURY & NEEDS CONSTANT OBSERVATION & CARE

DATE	TIME	NURSING ACTION	AMEND ACTION TIME, DATE AND SIGN	CHILD/PARENT ACTION	SIGN PARENT AND NURSE
28/5/93	1930	* CONTINUOUS OBSERVATIONS OF HEART RATE, BLOOD PRESSURE, INTRA CRANIAL PRESSURE USING AN APPROPRIATE MONITOR & RECORD HOURLY			
		* RECORD CEREBRAL PERFUSION PRESSURE HOURLY			
		* OBSERVE PUPIL SIZE, EQUALNESS & REACTION TO LIGHT, HOURLY & RECORD			
		* AIM TO KEEP INTRA CRANIAL PRESSURE BELOW 15mmHg & CEREBRAL PERFUSION PRESSURE BETWEEN 50-90 mmHg			
		* NURSE ON A 35° HEAD UP TILT BY USING WEDGE OR ELEVATED HEAD OF BED BASE			
		* ENSURE INTRA CRANIAL PRESSURE TRANSDUCER IS LEVEL WITH THE BRIDGE OF DONNA'S NOSE BY USING THE SPIRIT LEVEL MANOMETER			
		* ENSURE DONNA'S HEAD IS KEPT IN ALIGNMENT WITH HER BODY			
		* INFORM MEDICAL STAFF OF ANY CHANGES/DETERIORATION IN VITAL SIGNS			C. BROWN

The signature of the parent indicates that this care plan has been negotiated

NURSING CARE PLAN

NAME	DONNA JONES		HOSPITAL NO.	963148		AGE 11 YEARS

ACTIVITY OF LIVING ... SAFETY

PROBLEM/NEED ... DONNA HAS A HEAD INJURY & NEEDS CONSTANT OBSERVATION & CARE

DATE	TIME	NURSING ACTION	AMEND ACTION TIME, DATE AND SIGN	CHILD/PARENT ACTION	SIGN PARENT AND NURSE
28/5/93	19.30	* ONE-TO-ONE NURSING			
		* ENSURE IDENTITY BRACELET IS WORN AT ALL TIMES			
		* SET ALARM LIMITS ON THE MONITORING EQUIPMENT AS AGREED WITH MEDICAL STAFF			
		* OBSERVE CANNULA SITES HOURLY FOR SIGNS OF DISCONNECTION & LEAKAGE, INFLAMMATION OR INFILTRATION INTO TISSUES. CHECK PRESSURES VIA THE IVAC PUMP			
		* CARE OF ARTERIAL LINE AS PER UNIT POLICY : - NURSE RIGHT ARM EXPOSED - OBSERVE COLOUR & CIRCULATION OF DONNA'S RIGHT ARM - IDENTIFY ARTERIAL LINE WITH RED TAPE - MAINTAIN ARTERIAL FLUSH AT 2 mls HOURLY & RECORD - INFORM MEDICAL STAFF OF ANY DETERIORATION/CHANGE IN DONNA'S RIGHT ARM eg. BLANCHING ON FLUSHING, DISCOLOURATION, POOR CAPILLARY RETURN.			C. BROWN.

The signature of the parent indicates that this care plan has been negotiated

Fig. 6.10 (facing page)
Case study 3: Nursing
Care Plan – safety.

NURSING CARE PLAN – PROGRESS UPDATE

NAME DONNA JONES		HOSPITAL NO 963.148		AGE 11 YEARS

DATE	TIME	ACTIVITY OF LIVING SAFETY .... PROBLEM/NEED DONNA NEEDS OBSERVATION	SIGN
28/5/93	20·30	OBSERVATIONS STABLE FOLLOWING INCREASE IN RATE OF SEDATION. INTRA CRANIAL PRESSURE 4-10 mmHg, CEREBRAL PERFUSION PRESSURE > 60 mmHg. PUPIL SIZE 1-2 mm (FOLLOWING INCREASE IN SEDATION) + FAIRLY BRISK REACTION TO LIGHT. INTRAVENOUS CANNULA PATENT, PRESSURES VIA IVAC PUMPS LOW < 50 mmHg. RIGHT HAND WELL PERFUSED, GOOD CAPILLARY RETURN, ARTERIAL LINE SAMPLING + TRACING WELL.	C. BROWN

Fig. 6.11 Case study 3: Progress Update – safety.

NURSING CARE PLAN

NAME DONNA JONES		HOSPITAL NO 963148		AGE 11 YEARS

ACTIVITY OF LIVING EATING & DRINKING .... PROBLEM/NEED DONNA IS UNABLE TO EAT OR DRINK

DATE	TIME	NURSING ACTION	AMEND ACTION TIME, DATE AND SIGN	CHILD/PARENT ACTION	SIGN PARENT AND NURSE
28/5/93	19·30	* NIL BY MOUTH			
		* ADMINISTER PRESCRIBED INTRAVENOUS INFUSION			
		* MAINTAIN HOURLY FLUID BALANCE CHART - OBSERVING OVERALL BALANCE			
		* GIVE MOUTHCARE 2 HOURLY - OBSERVING CONDITION OF THE MOUTH		FOLLOWING INSTRUCTION LINDA + TONY WILL GIVE MOUTH CARE EVERY 2 HOURS WHEN PRESENT	T. JONES L. JONES
		* GIVE PRESCRIBED SUCRALFATE			
		* RECORD BLOOD SUGAR LEVELS 4-6 HOURLY			C. BROWN

The signature of the parent indicates that this care plan has been negotiated

Fig. 6.12 Case study 3: Nursing Care Plan – eating and drinking.

NURSING CARE PLAN – PROGRESS UPDATE

NAME DONNA JONES		HOSPITAL NO 963148		AGE 11 YEARS

DATE	TIME	ACTIVITY OF LIVING EATING + DRINKING ...... PROBLEM/NEED DONNA IS UNABLE TO EAT OR DRINK	SIGN
28/5/93	20·45	INTRAVENOUS HYDRATION MAINTAINED, MOUTHCARE GIVEN. MOUTH CLEAN & MOIST. BLOOD SUGARS STABLE 3·5 - 5·2 mmols	C. BROWN

Fig. 6.13 Case study 3: Progress Update – eating and drinking.

NURSING CARE PLAN

NAME	DONNA JONES		HOSPITAL NO. 963148		AGE 11 YEARS
ACTIVITY OF LIVING EMOTIONAL / SPIRITUAL			PROBLEM/NEED	DONNA IS CRITICALLY ILL & BOTH DONNA & HER PARENTS REQUIRE CLEAR EXPLANATIONS & EMOTIONAL SUPPORT	

DATE	TIME	NURSING ACTION	AMEND ACTION TIME, DATE AND SIGN	CHILD/PARENT ACTION	SIGN PARENT AND NURSE
28/5/93	19:00	* INTRODUCE SELF & OTHER MEMBERS OF STAFF TO DONNA & HER FAMILY			
		* SHOW DONNA'S PARENTS AROUND THE UNIT & ARRANGE ACCOMODATION IN THE PARENTS UNIT	28/5/93 20:00 C. BROWN		
		* CONTACT FAMILY CARE ASSISTANT TO ARRANGE MEAL VOUCHERS			
		* CONTACT THE HOSPITAL PRIEST FOR SPIRITUAL SUPPORT & PROVIDE A QUIET AREA FOR THE FAMILY TO EXPRESS THEIR FEELINGS IN PRIVACY	28/5/93 19:00 C. BROWN	LINDA & TONY WILL ASK FOR TOM DREW TO BE CONTACTED AS THEY WISH	L. JONES T. JONES
		* ALLOW & SUPPORT DONNA'S PARENTS TO EXPRESS THEIR FEELINGS REGARDING HER CONDITION			
		* EXPLAIN ALL PROCEDURES TO DONNA & HER PARENTS		LINDA & TONY WILL ASK QUESTIONS OR ASK TO SPEAK TO A DOCTOR WHENEVER THEY WISH	L. JONES T. JONES
		* KEEP DONNA'S PARENTS INFORMED ABOUT HER CONDITION & PROGRESS			
		* PROVIDE OPPORTUNITIES FOR DONNA'S PARENTS TO ASK ADDITIONAL QUESTIONS & ANSWER ANY QUERIES THEY HAVE, REFERRING TO THE NURSE IN CHARGE OR DOCTOR AS REQUIRED			
					C. BROWN
			The signature of the parent indicates that this care plan has been negotiated		

NURSING CARE PLAN

NAME	DONNA JONES		HOSPITAL NO. 963148		AGE 11 YEARS
ACTIVITY OF LIVING EMOTIONAL / SPIRITUAL			PROBLEM/NEED	DONNA IS CRITICALLY ILL & BOTH DONNA & HER PARENTS REQUIRE CLEAR EXPLANATIONS & EMOTIONAL SUPPORT	

DATE	TIME	NURSING ACTION	AMEND ACTION TIME, DATE AND SIGN	CHILD/PARENT ACTION	SIGN PARENT AND NURSE
28/5/93	19:00	IN CONJUNCTION WITH DONNA'S PARENTS, DEVISE A STIMULATION PROGRAMME FOR DONNA, & ENCOURAGE THEM TO TOUCH & TALK TO HER		LINDA & TONY WILL TOUCH & TALK TO DONNA, REASSURING HER, SHOW HER PHOTOGRAPHS, READ HER STORIES & PLAY HER FAVOURITE MUSIC CASSETTES. MATERNAL GRANDPARENTS WILL BRING IN HER FAVOURITE DOLLS & GAMES, & HER OWN BED CLOTHES	L. JONES T. JONES
					C. BROWN
			The signature of the parent indicates that this care plan has been negotiated		

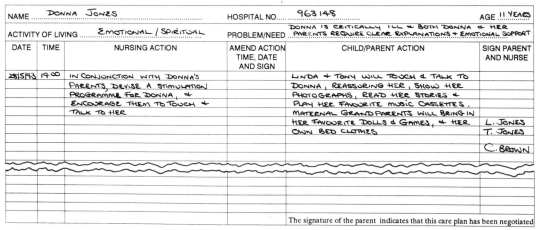

Fig. 6.14 Case study 3: Nursing Care Plan – emotional/spiritual.

NURSING CARE PLAN – PROGRESS UPDATE

NAME DONNA JONES		HOSPITAL NO 963148	AGE 11 YEARS	
DATE	TIME	ACTIVITY OF LIVING EMOTIONAL/SPIRITUAL PROBLEM/NEED DONNA & HER PARENTS NEED EMOTIONAL SUPPORT		SIGN
28/5/93	19.00	TOM DREW (RIC PRIEST) CONTACTED. WILL VISIT PICU TO SPEAK WITH		
		DONNA'S PARENTS		C.BROWN
	20.00	ACCOMODATION ARRANGED IN THE PARENTS UNIT FOR DONNA'S PARENTS		C.BROWN

Fig. 6.15 Case study 3: Progress Update – emotional/spiritual.

Fig 6.16 A nurse and parent delivering care in partnership.

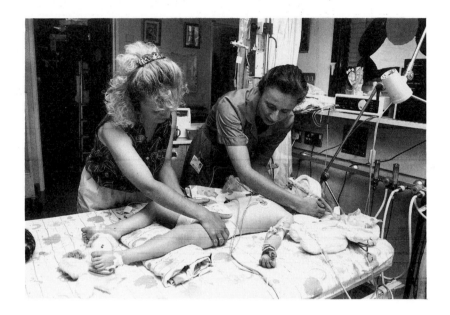

Part 3
Extending the Model

Introduction

The following chapters focus upon the application of key concepts of the model within specific settings and situations. Specifically-designed nursing records have been devised in order to:

- Acknowledge the nature of the work and workload in different settings.
- Overcome time-consuming difficulties associated with the completion of nursing records.
- Enable the nurse to quickly gather important and relevant information without compromising the philosophy or principles upon which the model is based.
- Enhance communication with other health care professionals. For example, the Theatre Checklist communicates information to theatre personnel, thereby enabling a child to continue to receive care which is not only safe but also geared towards meeting the child's needs as an individual.

Whilst a child's safety needs are addressed throughout, the development of a Theatre Checklist and Core Care Plans assist in enhancing this particular aspect of care.

Chapter 7
Caring for a Child and Family within an Accident and Emergency Department

Attendance at an Accident and Emergency (A & E) department is often the first and in many instances the only experience children have of a hospital environment. Muller *et al*. [1] indicate that by the age of five years, 44% of all children have sustained an injury that requires care and treatment at an Accident and Emergency department. Indeed, children account for up to 25% and in some instances one-third of all attendees at A & E departments [2]. However, many hospitals still do not provide separate facilities nor specialist staff to cater for the specific needs of children and their families. In view of the latter the approach to care often excludes the involvement of the child's carers in the care that the child receives during his/her visit.

The Department of Health document *Welfare of Children and Young People in Hospital* [3] states that within Accident and Emergency departments, '... appropriate provision is necessary to meet the needs of children and their families.' The ideal is the provision of specific and entirely separate Accident and Emergency facilities which cater purely for children. However, other Accident and Emergency departments can develop and enhance facilities offered for children and their families, and promote a child and family focused approach to care. In particular, attention must be given towards:

- Providing separate waiting areas with play and separate examination/treatment areas appropriately decorated and equipped for the needs of a child and family.
- Involving the child's parents and family in their child's care, facilitating and supporting their presence even within resuscitation areas if they wish.
- Developing effective policies and protocols for the care of children, including those related to the assessment of priorities for care/treatment and as a means to ensure that children receive care promptly and efficiently.
- Employing nursing staff who are specifically trained and experienced to meet a child and family's needs, thereby ensuring a child and family focused approach to care.

In view of the importance attached to prioritizing a child's need for care, the unpredictability of the workload within Accident and Emergency departments, and the time-consuming task of completing nursing records, the following documentation which reflects the needs of children and their families has been devised. The use of the documentation enhances the care that children and families receive, particularly in relation to the child's requirement for pain relief and the need to ensure that children and their families receive preparation for forthcoming procedures and events. Its use also ensures that care requirements, care delivery and information given to the child and family is communicated between all medical and nursing staff working within the department. This thereby ensures that the whole approach to care does not become fragmented and that the caring process is co-ordinated.

The Children's Accident and Emergency Nursing Documentation

The documentation (Fig. 7.1) reflects the philosophy of the Children's Unit, as well as the principles upon which all the nursing records are based (see chapter 2). The design of the documentation is based upon a systematic problem-solving approach involving assessment, implementation and review of care and progress update. If the child is admitted, a carbon copy of the documentation provides the nurse on the ward with information concerning the initial assessment made on arrival in the department, as well as details of all care given.

Guidelines

The initial assessment is based upon a tick box approach, thereby allowing the triage nurse to quickly document his/her assessment of the child's condition on arrival. Particular issues or problems may be enlarged upon as necessary in the history section of the documentation.

Triage categories

(1)	Life threatening	Children who need to be seen *immediately*, e.g. respiratory arrest, patients who are having convulsions.
(2)	Urgent	Those children who need to be seen by a doctor as soon as possible but who could safely wait up to *ten minutes*, e.g. asthmatics requiring a nebulizer, obvious fractures.
(3)	Can wait (1)	All other children presenting with a condition or injury appropriate to the A & E department.
(4)	Can wait (2)	Children for whom appropriate treatment/advice is available elsewhere, i.e. GP/health visitor.

A child's condition may alter following initial assessment. This should be noted in the Progress Update section and the triage category altered accordingly (see example below).

Children's Unit
Accident & Emergency Nursing Documentation

Life Threatening	Accompanied by
Urgent	
Can Wait (1)	Who has Parental
Can Wait (2)	Responsibility?

Next of Kin

In Dept
Aware
Not Aware
Need to Contact
Contacted

MOBILITY
- Mobile
- Restricted Mobility
- Imobile
- N/A

ASSESSMENT

BREATHING
| Spontaneous | | Wheezy | | Stridor |
| Irregular | | Apnoeic | | Recession/Nasal Flaring |

COLOUR
| Pink/Normal Colour | | Mottled | | Pale |
| Cyanosed | | | | |

COMMUNICATION
| Chatty/Babbling | | Crying | | Talking Normally |
| Not Speaking | | Shy/quiet | | Unconscious |

Problem:

SAFETY
Alert		Disorientated		Concious
Asleep/rousable		Irritable		Drowsy/rousable
Unconscious		Unresponsive		

0   20   40   60   80   100

COMFORT
Not in Pain		Generally Fractious/Miserable
In Pain		Location
Severe/Moderate/Slight		Duration

PAIN RELIEF/ANTIPYRETIC   YES/NO
Type   Last Dose
How   Dosage

OTHER MEDICATION   None

Allergies:

R   L

INJURY SITE AS SHOWN

L   R

CONTROL OF BODY TEMPERATURE
| Cold Extremities | | Feels Hot |
| Skin feels normal body temperature | | Flushed |

EATING & DRINKING
| Last Drink | Type | Problems: YES/NO/NA |
| Last Ate | NBM YES/NO | |

ELIMINATION
| Last passed Urine | | Problems: YES/NO/NA |
| Bowels | | Problems: YES/NO/NA |

EMOTIONAL/SPIRITUAL   N/A

WT			HT	
T	R	Oxygen Saturation	Peak Flow	
			PRE	POST
P	B/P	Urinalysis	BM	
		PERL YES/NO		

8   7   6   5   4   3   2   1

CARE OF SKIN
Skin intact
Skin not intact
Only visible areas examined
N/A

Example

Life threatening	10.30 AM
Urgent	
Can wait (1)	10.00 AM
Can wait (2)	

Child has febrile convulsion in the department.

Child with temperature who has been given paracetamol before arrival in the department.

Fig. 7.1 (left and right) The Children's Accident and Emergency Nursing Documentation.

History	Other Relevant Information
Signature Date Time	
Initial Care	Plan of Care
Given by Time	Given by Time

Time	Progress Update	Signature

OBSERVATIONS

Time								
Temp								
Pulse								
Resps								
B/P								

ADMISSION
Hospital Booklet
Bed Arranged
Bed Bureau
Nurse Escort
Porters Arranged

DISCHARGE
Medication
Advice Given
Information Leaflets
Type of leaflet........................
....
Ref. to Health Visitor   Y/N
Ref. to Social Worker
Parent Held Records
Transport arranged
if necessary

FOR FOLLOW UP
Appointment
No Follow–Up necessary
Directions
Transport Arranged If Necessary

Personal details

Accompanied by   Name(s) – first and surname.
Relationship to the child – the child may be brought to the A & E Department by someone other than the next-of-kin.

Next-of-kin   Name(s) – first and surname.
Document whether:

- they are present
- aware of the accident/visit
- need to be contacted
- contacted.

If the child is accompanied by someone other than a person with parental responsibility, the triage nurse or the person accompanying the child must contact the next-of-kin or another relative. In the event that a parent with parental responsibility is unable to travel to the department, consent to treatment may be obtained over the telephone. The name, relationship of the person contacted, time and details of the conversation must be documented in the Progress Update section of the documentation. If a person with parental responsibility cannot be contacted the triage nurse must record that attempts have been made to do so in the Progress Update section of the document.

Who has parental responsibility?   (See page 59.)

Who can acquire it?   (See page 60.)

Assessment
The appropriate box representing the clinical condition of the child should be ticked. It should be noted that a full assessment of certain Activities of Living will not always be appropriate, e.g. a child presenting with a minor cut to a finger will not require a full assessment of 'Eating/ Drinking'. However, every child should have an assessment of the following:

- breathing
- communication
- safety
- comfort

The appropriate face on the pain scale must also be ticked. Where possible children should indicate this themselves (Fig. 7.2). Problems/needs should be recorded in the relevant section where space allows, otherwise details should be documented in the 'History' or 'Other Information' section.

Pain relief/antipyretic   Record details of pain relief/antipyretic given prior to arrival in the department, including information concerning the usual method of administration, e.g. syrup via spoon.

Other medication   Record details of any other medication the child has been taking, e.g. antibiotics, including details of the dose, type and the time the last dose was given.

Emotional/spiritual   Record, if appropriate, religion, the need for support or counselling (parental or child).

Mobility/care of skin   Tick the appropriate box corresponding to the child's condition, with the diagrams being used to identify:

Fig. 7.2 A child using the Pain Scale to indicate her level of discomfort.

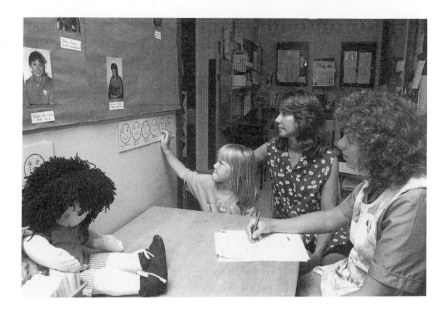

- the area of restricted mobility
- the site of: rashes
  lacerations
  contusions
  abrasions
  suspected fractures/bone deformity
  bruises
  swelling, etc.

If assessment of body temperature, eating and drinking, elimination or emotional/spiritual is considered to be inappropriate, the nurse must tick or record Not applicable in the appropriate section. All other areas must be completed.

Observations
The appropriate observations (dependent upon the child's condition) should be recorded. PERL (Pupils Equal and Reacting to Light), Yes/No/ Not applicable – delete or circle as appropriate and tick pupil size.

History
Record briefly details of illness or accident. The history should be taken if possible from the child, as well as the person accompanying the child.

Other relevant information
Record details of any other information that may affect the child and his/ her treatment, e.g. parents also involved in accident or the child is a known asthmatic/epileptic/haemophiliac.

Initial care

Details of any first-aid treatment should be recorded, e.g. saline packs to scald, sling applied, clean/irrigate wound, wash hair; baseline observations – weight, temperature, pulse, respiration, blood pressure, oxygen saturation, urinalysis, etc.

Plan of care

Record details of the plan of nursing intervention/action, e.g. administer antipyretic/pain relief and monitor effectiveness; observe for signs of haemorrhage – record pulse and blood pressure every 15 minutes.

The triage nurse must also document whether the child has been referred to a Nurse Practitioner or Senior House Officer and, in the event that the child is not accompanied by a person with parental responsibility, whether a person with parental responsibility needs to be contacted. Parents/carers should be asked to sign the plan of care when they have agreed to undertake aspects of care, thereby denoting that care has been discussed and negotiated with them (see chapter 5). For example:

- When a urine sample is required and parents agree to collect or supervize collection.
- When sedation has been administered prior to treatment and the parents subsequently agree to observe the child and to inform their nurse when the child is asleep/drowsy.

Progress update

Record details of the outcome of care given or changes in condition. In respect of GP emergency referrals, the time the appropriate doctor is informed of the child's arrival must be documented. It is important that each entry is signed and the time recorded. The observation/fluid balance sections should also be used as and when appropriate.

Admission/discharge/follow-up section

Complete as appropriate. In the event that the child has been accompanied by someone other than a parent with parental responsibility, the nurse must follow the discharge policy and document in the Progress Update section the name and the relationship of the person with whom the child is discharged. Details of any information regarding follow-up care/treatment and the time of departure must also be recorded.

In the above instances (having first gained permission from the patient) details of diagnosis, treatment, advice (written advice leaflets, etc.) and follow-up care should be given in writing to the accompanying person, the social worker, or to the child him/herself for transmission to the person with parental responsibility. Whenever possible the nurse should discuss these details with the person with parental responsibility, if not in person then via the telephone.

If the child is unaccompanied, the nurse must follow the discharge policy related to unaccompanied children/young people.

References

1. Muller, D.J., Harris, P.J., Wattley, L. & Taylor, J.D. (1992) *Nursing Children: Psychology, research and practice.* Chapman & Hall, London.
2. British Paediatric Association, British Association of Paediatric Surgeons and Casualty Surgeons Association (1988) *Joint Statement on Children's Attendance at Accident & Emergency Departments.*
3. Department of Health (1991) *Welfare of Children and Young People in Hospital.* HMSO, London.

Chapter 8
Enabling Shorter Lengths of Stay

Day case surgery

The Department of Health document *Welfare of Children and Young People in Hospital* [1] states that children should be admitted, '...to hospital only if the care they require cannot be as well provided at home, in a day clinic or on a day basis in hospital.' In recent years there has been a considerable increase in the number of operations and procedures performed on a 'day case' basis [1–6]. The main driving forces behind this growth are related to changes in clinical practice, technological developments and financial pressures upon the NHS [3–5]. However, day case surgery offers considerable benefits for children, including the reduction in waiting lists and the provision of a better service organized and geared towards meeting children's needs. Nevertheless, the considerable interest, particularly from managers, can perhaps be attributed to the enormous potential which day case surgery can offer in relation to the reduction of costs and increased patient throughput, all of which can improve an organization's economy, efficiency and effectiveness.

The benefits of day case surgery for the child and family are considerable, particularly in relation to the reduction in the amount of time the child spends in a strange and unfamiliar hospital environment and in the time the child is separated from the family, as well as their usual routine/activities. Day case surgery assists in preventing the detrimental psychological and emotional effects associated with longer hospital stays, facilitates the maintenance of the integrity of the family unit and enables the family to retain greater 'control' over their child's care and recovery [7].

The Day Case Sheet

In view of the considerable growth in day case surgery and the potential for further expansion, the Nottingham Children's Unit recognized the need to adapt the nursing records and produce a concise version, the Day Case Sheet (Fig. 8.1). This enables the nurse to quickly gather important and relevant information in order to provide care that reflects the specific needs of an individual child and family, without compromising the underlying principles and philosophy reflected within the model of care.

Guidelines

Introduction

This sheet is designed for children admitted as elective surgical day cases. These children will be admitted for less than 12 hours and accompanied by a parent or carer throughout the duration of their admission. The Day Case Sheet replaces the full nursing process records and incorporates a Theatre Checklist. It should be kept with the child throughout the admission.

The information should be obtained from the child and his/her parents or carers. The completion of the Day Case Sheet provides the ideal opportunity for a good rapport between the nurse, child and family to develop, during which time a two-way exchange of information occurs. It should be acknowledged that the family have the best knowledge of the child and they must therefore be involved from the outset. The Day Case Sheet must be completed by a qualified member of nursing staff. If subsequent information becomes known at a later stage this addition must be signed, dated and the time of its inclusion recorded. Any part of the Day Case Sheet that is not relevant should have 'Not applicable' inserted into the appropriate box. On the Theatre Checklist 'Not applicable' should be circled.

Personal details

Name, address and date of birth or 'sticky label'.

Likes to be called   The child's choice (if possible) – nickname or full name.

Who has parental responsibility?   (See page 59.)

Who can acquire it?   (See page 60.)

Time, date and proposed operation

State operation, procedure or investigation.

Ward facilities

The facilities available within the Unit (see list – Fig. 8.1) should be discussed and shown to families during the admission period. In order to ensure that *all* information has been given, the nurse must tick when this has been completed.

Special needs

Those aspects of care that are individual to the child, e.g. feeds, long lines and special hygiene needs, should be recorded here.

Observations/fluid section(s)

Record the relevant information following the operation, procedure or investigation.

DAY CASE SHEET

AFFIX THEATRE BAR CODE LABEL	CHECKLIST	WARD CIRCLE			CHECKLIST	WARD CIRCLE		
	Operation Gown & bath	N/A	Y	N	Completed notes		Y	N
	Jewellery removed	N/A	Y	N	X-rays	N/A	Y	N
	Make-up/nail varnish removed	N/A	Y	N	Sickle Cell result	N/A	Y	N
Date: Time:	Prothesis/contact lenses removed	N/A	Y	N	Parent & Nurse to accompany child		Y	N
Child's Name:					Toy/comforter accompanying		Y	N
Address:	Braces removed	N/A	Y	N	Removed sutures etc, wanted			
	Loose teeth	N/A	Y	N	by child	N/A	Y	N
Hospital No:	Capped crowned teeth	N/A	Y	N	Explanation of procedure to:			
Name(s) of Parent(s):	Identification				Child		Y	N
	bracelet checked	N/A	Y	N	Carer		Y	N
Likes to be called:	Allergy band	N/A	Y	N	Any phobia/anxiety		Y	N
Ward:	Consent signed		Y	N				
Consultant:	Pre-medication given	N/A	Y	N				
Proposed Operation:	Topical precannulation cream	N/A	Y	N	Special instruction/preparation		Y	N
Allergies: (write in red)	Theatre tag checked	N/A	Y	N				
	Fasted from:	Diet:						
		Fluid:						
	Pre-operative Observations							
Special needs relevant to theatre care:								
Likes to be called:								
Hospital Facilities – tick box when explained to parents								
Parents' Kitchen								
Parents' Sitting Room/Smoking Room								
Ward Kitchen								
Parent Information Board/file								
Parent shower/toilet facilities					Ward Nurse Signature:			
Telephone								
Dining room facilities					Date: Time:			

Discharge section
(See page 61.)

If the child is to remain in hospital overnight, the 'Shared Medical and Nursing Short Stay Admission Sheet' must be used. If hospital care continues for more than 24 hours the full nursing process records must be completed.

Ward communication

The time the child returns to the ward, as well as details that acknowledge handover between nursing staff and Progress Update, should be recorded. It is important from a legal viewpoint that the nurse records the date and time and signs any entry made in this section.

Short stay medical admissions

Local and national statistics highlight that although the number of children admitted to hospital has increased, the length of stay has steadily declined over recent years [2]. This reflects not only advances in relation to care, but also the fact that the central focus of the caring process is upon involving the child's parents and family at a much earlier stage. The emphasis is towards teaching and supporting them to adapt and develop additional caring skills, thereby facilitating earlier discharge from hospital. In addition,

Fig. 8.1 (left and right)
The Day Case Sheet.

Nottingham Children's Unit Day Case Sheet

Operation or procedure Performed

Special instructions/problems/comments:-

Analgesia given:

Ward communication:	Time warded:	Assessment of Pain:

Trained Nurse signature:-

OBSERVATIONS					FLUIDS				
Time								Output	
Temp					Time	Intake	Urine	Vomit	Other
Pulse									
Resp									
B.P.									
Wound									
Other									

DISCHARGE INFORMATION

G.P. Letter: Patient held records: seen
                                                                  completed

Appt: Ward
             Clinic
             Other
                                     Advice given:
Medicines T.T.O. given

                                     Parent Information Leaflets:

                                     Time of Discharge:

                                     Signature:

                                     Date:

earlier discharge planning, improved liaison with health care professionals in the community and the development of paediatric community nursing teams to provide continued support at home have assisted in this process [see Part 4].

The rapid throughput of children (many of whom are admitted for less than 24 hours) led to the development of a Short Stay Admission Sheet which substantially reduces the time spent upon completing paperwork. The Shared Medical and Nursing Short Stay Admission Sheet reflects:

● The principles and philosophy upon which the model of care is based.
● The increasing move towards the sharing of information and collaboration between health care professionals.
● The need for early discharge planning and liaison between hospital-based and community-based health care professionals.

The Shared Medical and Nursing Short Stay Admission Sheet

The Shared Medical and Nursing Short Stay Admission Sheet (Fig. 8.2) has been designed to eliminate excessive and time-consuming paperwork for both nurses and doctors for a short admission. The Short Stay Admission Sheet reflects the philosophy of the Unit and the principles upon which all the nursing records are based.

Criteria for use

● The child's mother/father or usual carer should be resident and remain within the hospital for the duration of the admission.
● It is anticipated that the child will be admitted and discharged within a 24-hour-period.
● The Shared Medical and Nursing Short Stay Admission Sheet can be utilized for all planned or emergency admissions provided that they meet the above criteria.

Guidelines

Introduction
The Short Stay Admission Sheet is intended to be a *shared* record between nurses and medical staff. The use of the Short Stay Admission Sheet should be a joint decision between the doctor and an experienced nurse. During use it is preferable for the sheet to be kept by the child's bedside, as is the case with all other nursing records. However, following discharge it is *essential* that it is filed in the correct chronological sequence in the child's medical notes. It should not be filed with other nursing charts/records in the back of the notes.

History Sheet
This is a concise version of the History Sheet that is incorporated into the full nursing process records and therefore the appropriate guidelines should be followed (see chapter 3). Details concerning previous admissions/health problems should be recorded on a Communication Sheet as appropriate and the nurse completing the History Sheet *must* sign in the appropriate space. The allergies and current medication section may be completed by the nursing or medical staff.

Medical information
This section is completed as appropriate by the medical staff caring for the child.

Nursing information

'On Admission Assessment' section   Those Activities of Living that are considered to be the most appropriate to a short stay admission have been

included in this section. This is *not* an assessment of the child's usual routine. Any queries concerning the child's norm can be clarified with the carer resident with the child. This section should be used to highlight the child's problems/needs on admission. For example, if the child was feverish this would be recorded in the 'Care of Skin/Body Temperature' section, whereas if the child had ingested shampoo this would be noted in 'Safety'.

Further *examples* of the kind of information and observations that may be recorded in this section can be found in chapter 3. The child's height, weight and urinalysis should be recorded in the appropriate box situated in the assessment grid. The nurse completing the On Admission Assessment grid *must* date, time and sign in the appropriate boxes.

Care Plan

There is space for two problems/needs within the Care Plan section of the Short Stay Admission Sheet. However, an additional sheet (Fig. 8.3) is available if the child has more than two needs/problems.

The first two columns of the Care Plan should be completed as instructed in chapter 4. However, instead of having separate 'Nursing Action' and 'Child/Parent Action' columns, care should be prescribed in the 'Action' column and the 'Nurse' or 'Parent' column ticked according to who will carry out each action. This should be negotiated between the nurse and child or parent as care is planned (see chapter 4), the child and/or parent (as appropriate) being asked to sign the Care Plan to document that they agree with the information that has been recorded. The signatures *do not* suggest that the parents are taking responsibility for their child's care but that the Care Plan is a true record of the nurse, parent and child negotiated plan of care. It should be noted that some parents may choose not to sign.

Progress Update

The care planned in the 'Action' column should be reviewed and updated at least once during each shift. Details concerning the implementation and continuation of care, as well as a review of the outcomes of the care provided, should be recorded in the 'Progress Update' section.

'Observation' section

The child's initial observations on admission should be recorded in the first column. However, it is also important that the time is recorded. The two blank columns can be used to record other observations, e.g. blood glucose, oxygen saturation readings, etc. Neurological observations should be recorded on the appropriate neurological observation chart as the scope of this sheet is inadequate to record all the necessary information.

'Fluids' section

The column marked 'Other' can be used to record urinalysis, bowel actions or other relevant information as appropriate to the individual child.

MEDICAL INFORMATION

Examination

Diagnosis

Investigations

Plan

Review

NOTTINGHAM CHILDREN'S UNIT
SHARED NURSING/MEDICAL
SHORT STAY ADMISSION SHEET

HISTORY SHEET

Hospital No:

Name: Date: Time:

Age: HV:

Who has parental responsibility   Address:
for the child?:

Who accompanies the child?:

                               Allergies:

Medical Diagnosis: Current Medication:

Reason for admission: Recent Contact with infectious diseases:

Why do the parents think the child   Ward facilities - tick box when explained
has been admitted?:   to parents:
                                       Parents' Kitchen
                                       Parents' Sitting/Smoking Room
                                       Ward Kitchen
Why does the child think he/she   Parent Information Board/File
has been admitted?:   Parent Shower/Toilet Facilities
                                       Canteen/Eating Facilities
                                       Telephone
Parents perception of previous admission: Fire Regulations explained   Yes/No
                                       Parents resident
                                       Where:
                                       Likes to be known as:

Named Nurse: Signature:

Date: Time:

MEDICAL INFORMATION

History

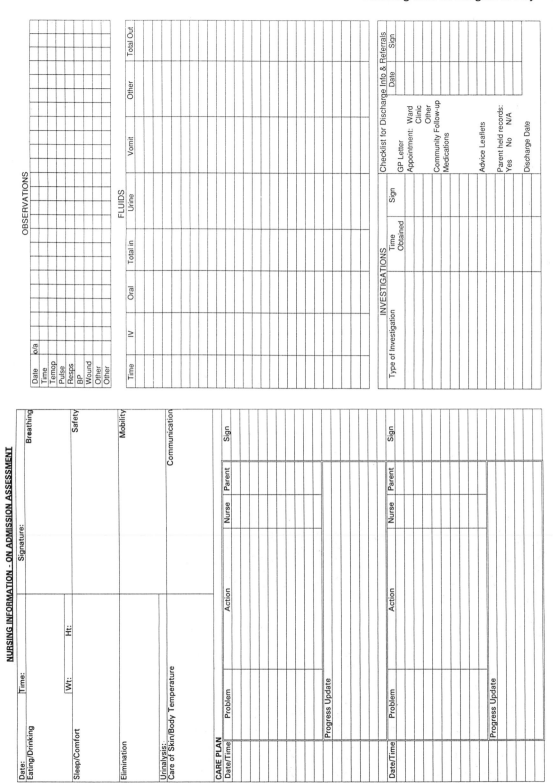

Fig. 8.2 The Shared Medical and Nursing Short Stay Admission Sheet.

Fig. 8.3 Short Stay, Shared Care Continuation Sheet.

SHORT STAY, SHARED CARE CONTINUATION SHEET

Hospital No:			Name:			
Ward:			Consultant:			

NURSING CARE PLAN

Date/Time	Problem	Action	Nurse	Parent	Sign
	Progress Update				
Date/Time	Problem	Action	Nurse	Parent	Sign
	Progress Update				
Date/Time	Problem	Action	Nurse	Parent	Sign
	Progress Update				

Investigations

The purpose of this section is to ensure that investigations or procedures are carried out efficiently, safely and at the correct time. The type of investigation required and the time it is to be performed should be documented in the appropriate boxes, e.g. paracetamol blood levels following ingestion, times of blood samples during a glomerular filtration rate (GFR) test, times of x-rays or scans. There is also a column to be ticked when the investigation has been completed. Some investigations/specimens will not require the time to be recorded, but the column will need to be ticked once they have been performed or obtained. The nurse must sign when the investigations/specimens have been performed or obtained and sent to the relevant laboratory.

'Discharge information/referral' section

The named nurse caring for the child will take responsibility for completing this section before discharge. The relevant boxes should be ticked and signed as appropriate. Although this section tends to be completed by nursing staff, medical staff are encouraged to complete relevant sections of the check list as appropriate, e.g. GP letter, ward appointment and medications.

References

1. Department of Health (1991) *Welfare of Children and Young People in Hospital.* HMSO, London.
2. Audit Commission (1993) *Children First: A Study of Hospital Services.* HMSO, London.
3. Audit Commission (1990) *A Short Cut to Better Services.* HMSO, London.
4. Audit Commission (1991) *Measuring Quality: The Patient's View of Day Surgery.* NHS Occasional Paper **3**, HMSO, London.
5. Audit Commission (1992) *All in a Day's Work: An Audit of Day Surgery in England and Wales.* NHS Occasional Paper **4**, HMSO, London.
6. Trent Regional Health Authority (1990) *Children and Young People Services Statistical Tables for 1988/1989.* Trent Regional Health Authority, Sheffield.
7. Caring for Children in the Health Services (1991) *Just For The Day.* CCHS, Bristol.

Chapter 9
Promoting Safety: A Theatre Checklist and Core Care Plans

The Theatre Checklist

The Theatre Checklist (Fig. 9.1) has been devised to enable the nurse to quickly document important and essential information about a child which needs to be known by theatre personnel in order that they may be able to provide care which is safe and meets the child's individual needs. The Theatre Checklist reflects the philosophy of the Unit and the principles underpinning the model of care. The child and family's needs are addressed by sections such as:

- 'Child/parents prepared for High Dependency area'
- 'Parent and nurse to accompany child
- 'Toy/comforter accompanying'
- 'Explanation of procedure to child/carer'

CHILDREN'S UNIT PRE–OPERATIVE THEATRE CHECKLIST

AFFIX BAR CODE LABEL

Date: Time:

Child's Name:
Address:

Hospital No:

Ward:

Consultant:

Proposed Operation:

Allergies: (write in red)

Special needs relevant to theatre care:

Pre–operative Observations
T   P   R   BP   Cuff Size   Limb

Weight   Urinalysis

CHECKLIST	WARD CIRCLE			THEATRE CIRCLE			CHECKLIST	WARD CIRCLE		
Operation Gown & bath	N/A	Y	N	N/A	Y	N	Completed notes		Y	N
Jewellery removed	N/A	Y	N	N/A	Y	N	X–rays	N/A	Y	N
Make–up/nail varnish removed	N/A	Y	N	N/A	Y	N	Sickle Cell result	N/A	Y	N
Prothesis/contact lenses removed	N/A	Y	N	N/A	Y	N	Child/parents prepared for High Dependency area	N/A	Y	N
							Parent & Nurse to accompany child		Y	N
Braces removed	N/A	Y	N	N/A	Y	N	Toy/comforter accompanying		Y	N
Loose teeth	N/A	Y	N	N/A	Y	N	Removed sutures etc, wanted by child	N/A	Y	N
Capped crowned teeth	N/A	Y	N	N/A	Y	N				
Identification bracelet checked	N/A	Y	N	N/A	Y	N	Explanation of procedure to: Child		Y	N
Allergy band	N/A	Y	N	N/A	Y	N	Carer		Y	N
Consent signed		Y	N		Y	N	Any phobia/anxiety		Y	N
Pre–medication given	N/A	Y	N	N/A	Y	N				
Topical precannulation cream	N/A	Y	N	N/A	Y	N				
Theatre tag checked	N/A	Y	N	N/A	Y	N				
Fasted from: Time / Diet / Fluids							Special instruction/preparation		Y	N

KEY: N/A = Not Applicable
     Y = YES
     N = NO

Theatre Nurse Signature:
Date: Time:

Ward Nurse Signature:
Date: Time:

Guidelines

Each box of the Theatre Checklist must be completed. The bar code label is affixed (to the top left-hand corner) by theatre personnel.

Side 1

Special needs relevant to theatre care For example, allergies, hearing or speech problems, physical or mental handicaps, previous anaesthetic problems, plaster of paris *in situ*, catheter,colostomy, ileostomy, central venous line *in situ*, medical conditions and special treatments, need to be described in order to maintain good communication and safety when transferring a child to theatre. Circle appropriate Yes/No/Not Applicable response in column. Theatres to complete according to their protocol.

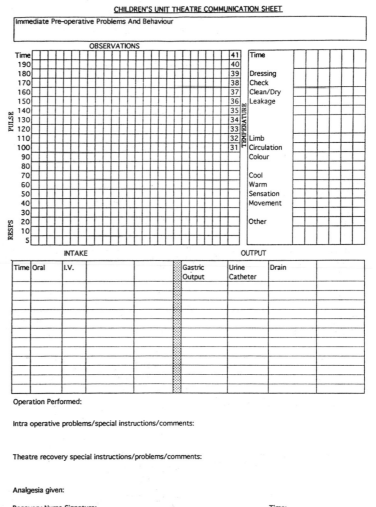

Fig. 9.1 (left and right) The Theatre Checklist.

Fasted from   Insert appropriate 'fast from' times for diet and fluids, as sometimes they are different.

Phobia/anxiety   Describe any specific problems and communicate these to the theatre nurse, e.g. needle phobia, anaesthetic mask, parental separation, fear of being awake, etc.

Special instruction/preparation   For example, bowel washout given prior to theatre, limb elevation, catheterization, position of intravenous cannulae, to ensure that special instructions and specific preparation have been followed and documented.

Ward nurse's signature   The ward nurse must sign the Theatre Checklist immediately prior to the child leaving the ward.

Side 2

Immediate pre-operative problems/behaviour   Record by theatre nurse of child's emotional state/behaviour immediately prior to theatre, e.g. sleeping, crying, screaming, anxious, etc.

Observation section   Commence the recording of observations, e.g. temperature, pulse, respiration, wound and limb, in theatre. In short stay children, this sheet may continue to be used on the ward.

Dressings/circulation section   The time should be inserted in the top column and the appropriate box ticked. Any comments should be recorded in the 'Theatre recovery special instructions/problems/comments' section. On the ward it may be necessary to commence another chart for observation of 'Other' problems, e.g. reddened/broken areas. It is important to ensure that problems are clearly labelled.

Intake/output section   Commence observation and fluid charts in theatre and continue in the ward area if appropriate.

Theatre notes section   To be completed in theatre:

- Operation performed
- Intra operative problems
- Recovery problems
- Analgesia given
- Observation of wound or limb circulation.

Core Care Plans

Many nurses throw up their hands in horror when the topic of producing Core Care Plans is mentioned. It is feared that these may not only be abused but also that individuality and creativity could well be lost. However, Glasper *et al.* [1] indicate that a pre-written care plan should not be regarded as, '...a standardized plan of care which aims to make the patient fit the plan,' but one that incorporates agreed procedures, as well as crucial and immediate care, and decreases the process of continually rewriting the same information again and again. It is therefore increasingly being recognized that there is an occasional need in certain instances to have care plans written in a core format, for example pre- and post-operative care. These should, however, reflect both the philosophy of the unit and the principles upon which the nursing records are based.

It is important to ensure that any care plan is written so as to ensure that care is appropriately geared towards meeting the individual child's needs. However, sometimes a compromise has to be made in order to allow the nurse as much time as possible to care for the child and family. Core Care Plans, when used appropriately, assist in this process. They are a means of producing a clear and concise plan of care to guide nursing practice [2].

When producing Core Care Plans they must:

● Have the facility to be individualized for the special needs of each child and family.
● Be written in a standard format which reflects the Nottingham model.
● Be rationalized, research based and reviewed regularly so as to ensure accuracy and relevance.
● Be written and reviewed by RSCNs and other members of the health care team as appropriate.
● Be validated by the Nursing Process Working Group so as to ensure that all of the above is maintained.

Some examples of core care plans, which may be used as a base on which to plan individual care, include:

● Pre-anaesthetic care: safety
● Pre-operative and Pre-procedural: emotional
● Pre- and Post-procedure: safety
● Post-anaesthetic care: safety

Pre-anaesthetic care: safety (Fig. 9.2)

Guidelines

(1) Insert child's name, hospital number and age.
(2) Complete 'Problem/Need' statement by inserting the child's name.
(3) Insert date and time.

Nursing Action column

(4) Insert the time from which the child should be 'nil by mouth'.
(5) Ensure that care specific to the individual child is recorded.

Amend Action: Date, Time and Sign column

(6) Record changes and complete details concerning nursing action as appropriate.

		PAEDIATRIC NURSING CORE CARE PLAN			
		PRE ANAESTHETIC CARE (SAFETY)			
NAME		HOSPITAL NO.		AGE	
ACTIVITY OF LIVING ....SAFETY .... PROBLEM/NEED ....is having a general anaesthetic and needs to be safely cared for pre-anaesthetic					
DATE	TIME	NURSING ACTION PRE ANAESTHETIC CARE	AMEND ACTION Date Time & Sign	CHILD/PARENT ACTION	SIGN PARENT AND NURSE
		* Record base line observation of temp, pulse, respiratory rate and blood pressure. Report any abnormality to nurse in charge/doctor.			
		* Ensure that pre-medication has been prescribed to avoid delay.			
		* Ensure that cots sides are in situ to prevent falls.			
		* Record the time the doctor informed of arrival to avoid confusion.			
		* Ensure oxygen and suction are available and in working order, near to the bedside.			
		* Complete theatre checklist.			
		* Nil by mouth from			

Fig. 9.2 Core Care Plan: pre-anaesthetic care – safety.

(7) The nurse must sign and record the date and time of the above changes in this column.

Child/Parent Action column

(8) The plan of care should be discussed with the child, parents and family. The nurse should negotiate the degree of participation they wish to undertake with support, guidance and teaching. Specific measures, time and frequencies, etc. concerning their agreed level of involvement should be recorded in the 'Child/Parent Action' column.

(9) The negotiated plan should then be shown to the parents and family, so as to ensure that they understand and agree with the care that is recorded.

(10) Inform the child and parent/carer that care may be re-negotiated at any time (see chapter 5).

Signature column

(11) The child or parents should then be asked to sign the care plan signifying that they agree with the plan of care that has been shown to them. Their signature does not suggest that the child or parent is taking responsibility for this care but that the care plan has been shown and discussed with them.

(12) The nurse completing and negotiating the plan of care *must* sign the care plan.

Pre-operative and pre-procedural: emotional (Fig. 9.3)

(As for *Pre-anaesthetic care: safety* but not point (4) and with an additional point in the Child/Parent Action column.)

PAEDIATRIC NURSING CORE CARE PLAN					
PRE OPERATIVE AND PRE PROCEDURAL CARE (EMOTIONAL)					
NAME .... HOSPITAL NO. .... AGE					
ACTIVITY OF LIVING .... EMOTIONAL .... PROBLEM/NEED ....and family need clear explanations and support regarding the anaesthetic and procedure.					
DATE	TIME	NURSING ACTION PRE ANAESTHETIC CARE	AMEND ACTION Date Time & Sign	CHILD/PARENT ACTION	SIGN PARENT AND NURSE
		*Introduce self and other staff members to the child and family.			
		*Show around the ward areas and explain hospital facilities.			
		*Explain all procedures to child and family.			
		*Answer any questions and queries to try and allay anxiety referring on to nurse in charge/doctor if appropriate.			
		*Show appropriate video to help reduce stress if required.			
		*Organise theatre clothing for carer to accompany child to theatre.			

Fig. 9.3 Core Care Plan: pre-operative and pre-procedural – emotional.

Child/Parent Action column

(9) Any questions or queries answered by the nurse should be recorded in this column.

Pre- and post-procedure: safety (Fig. 9.4)

(As for *Pre-anaesthetic care: safety* except for the 'Nursing Action' column.)

Pre-procedure Nursing Action column

(4) Insert which base line observations are required.
(5) Insert the time that sedation should be given.
(6) Insert the time from which the child should be 'nil by mouth'.
(7) Insert the time the topical anaesthetic cream should be applied.
(8) Add any other individual nursing action required.

		PAEDIATRIC NURSING CORE CARE PLAN PRE AND POST PROCEDURAL CARE (SAFETY)			
NAME			HOSPITAL NO.		AGE ....
ACTIVITY OF LIVING ....safety........			PROBLEM/NEED .... is visiting the ward for .... (procedure) & requires pre and post safety care.		
DATE	TIME	NURSING ACTION PRE ANAESTHETIC CARE	AMEND ACTION Date Time & Sign	CHILD/PARENT ACTION	SIGN PARENT AND NURSE
		PRE PROCEDURE CARE			
		*Record baseline observation of ....and report any deviation from normal to nurse in charge/doctor.			
		*Ensure oxygen and suction are available and in working order, near to the bedside.			
		*Ensure that child is wearing an identity bracelet to avoid confusion.			
		*Record the time the doctor is informed of child's arrival & inform the family of any delays.			
		*Ensure that required sedation has been prescribed to avoid delays. Give sedation at .... hours.			
		*Ensure consent has been signed if required. If a general anaesthetic is required ensure child is nil by mouth from .... hours.			
		*If topical anaesthetic cream is required, apply at .... hours to reduce pain on cannulation.			
		POST PROCEDURE CARE			
		*Ensure airway is clear by checking breathing - report any problems to nurse in charge.			
		*Commence fluids when fully awake or as post procedure instructions.			
		*Ensure vomit bowls & tissues are available.			
		*Record observations of .... & report any deviation from normal to nurse in charge/doctor.			

Fig. 9.4 Core Care Plan: pre- and post-procedure – safety.

Post-procedure: Nursing Action column

(9)   Check post-procedure instructions and the child's ability to tolerate oral fluids prior to commencement.

(10)   Insert observations required.

(11)   Add any other individual nursing action required.

Post-anaesthetic care: safety (Fig. 9.5)

(As for *Pre-anaesthetic care: safety* except for the Nursing Action column.)

Nursing Action column

(4)   Insert observations required.

(5)   Record the frequency observations using specific times, e.g. half-hourly, hourly, etc.

(6)   Check the operation instructions and the child's ability to tolerate oral fluids prior to commencement.

(7)   Add any other individual nursing action required.

DATE	TIME	NURSING ACTION POST ANAESTHETIC CARE	AMEND ACTION Date Time & Sign	CHILD/PARENT ACTION	SIGN PARENT AND NURSE

PAEDIATRIC NURSING CORE CARE PLAN
POST ANAESTHETIC CARE (SAFETY)

NAME ....   HOSPITAL NO. ....   AGE ....

ACTIVITY OF LIVING   ....SAFETY .... PROBLEM/NEED ....is having a general anaesthetic and needs
to be cared for safely post-adeno/tonsillectomy.

Nursing actions:
* Ensure that child is fully rousable and that airway is clear by checking breathing pattern.
* Observe for colour alteration from his/her normal.
* Ensure oxygen and suction are available and in working order, near to the bedside.
* Record observations of pulse and respiration. Frequency: half hourly from ....hrs; 1 hourly from ....hrs; 4 hourly from ....hrs
* Record and report abnormalities to nurse in charge/doctor immediately.
* Observe for frequent swallowing and other signs of bleeding.
* Record BP if bleeding.
* Record 4 hourly temperature.
* Ensure cot sides are raised when unattended.
* Check and record when child is able to pass urine to ensure there are no problems.
* Wash and change into own clothes (when appropriate) to maintain comfort.

Fig. 9.5 Core Care Plan: post-anaesthetic care – safety.

Case study 4
William Clark: promoting safety through the use of a Theatre Checklist and Core Care Plans

The following case study demonstrates the application of the Nottingham model and a child and family focused approach to care. In particular, this case study highlights the use of Core Care Plans and the Theatre Checklist in order to ensure that a child's safety needs are met.

William, a two-year-old boy who likes to be known as Bobby, was admitted to Cedar ward for repair of glandular hypospadius. He was accompanied by his mother Jane Clark. On arrival they were greeted by staff nurse Paul Jones. Paul was to be Bobby's named nurse during his hospital stay.

It can be seen that in addition to highlighting the concept of negotiated care, the Core Care Plans have been individualized to reflect Bobby's needs (Figs 9.6–9.12). The importance of preparing Bobby and his mother for forthcoming events and procedures has been acknowledged within the plan of care. It should also be noted that Paul has explained to Jane (Bobby's mother) and Bobby that they can ask questions about the operation at any time. This indicates that Paul appreciates Bobby's and Jane's need to be given the opportunity to ask ques-

WARD: CEDAR	*CHILD'S HISTORY SHEET 1*		REG NO: 784892
Family Name: CLARK	Date: 7/9/93	Time: 10 AM	Family's perception of previous admission:
First Name: WILLIAM JOHN	Reason for admission:		MOTHER WAS IMPRESSED WHEN
Likes to be called: BOBBY	INCOMPLETE FORESKIN, SPRAYING		SHE VISITED A FRIEND'S CHILD
Age: 3 YRS	OF URINE		ON THE WARD ABOUT 6/12 AGO
DOB: 5-8-90	Accompanied by: MOTHER		
Birth weight: 8lb 1oz	Why do the parents think the child has		
Religion: C/E	been admitted:		
Child's Address: 29 RUSHWOOD CRESENT	TO CORRECT MILD DEFORMITY		Parent(s) Carer(s) Resident: YES/~~NO~~
ARNOLD	OF TIP OF PENIS		MOM
NOTTINGHAM			Where: BY BOBBY'S BED
Postcode: NG5 6SE	Medical Diagnosis:		Likes to be known as: JANE
	GLANDULAR HYPOSPADIAS		Do they wish to participate in the care of the child:
Telephone No: 469201			YES - EVERYDAY CHILD CARE
Next of Kin: JOHN & JANE CLARK	What reason does the child give for		
Relationship to child: PARENTS	this admission:		
Address if different from above:	TO MAKE HIM THE SAME		Social Arrangements:
AS ABOVE FOR MOTHER	AS OTHER LITTLE BOYS		MOTHER'S SISTER - AUNTIE CLARE
FATHER: 42 HIGH STREET			WILL BE CARING FOR TOM & ANNIE
BEESTON			AT HOME.
NOTTINGHAM			THEY WILL VISIT ON A DAILY BASIS,
NG9 3JN			AFTER TOM & ANNIE RETURN HOME
Telephone No: FATHER: 374861	Previous relevant history/admissions:		FROM SCHOOL
Work: DAD 368902 Home: MOTHER: 469201	HEALTHY LITTLE BOY WHO HAS NOT		
With whom does the child reside:	REQUIRED A PREVIOUS HOSPITAL		
JANE , TOM & ANNIE	ADMISSION		
Relationship to Child: MOTHER , BROTHER & SISTER			Name and age of siblings:
Who has parental responsibility			TOM - 8 YRS
for this child?: BOTH PARENTS			ANNIE - 5 YRS
MOTHER FATHER			
Telephone number: 469201 374861			
Child's Nurse/Team: PAUL JONES	Consultant: MR SCOTT		

Fig. 9.6 Case study 4: History Sheet 1.

tions at any time, thereby diminishing any fears or anxiety they have regarding the operation.

Paul's plan of care also addresses Bobby's and Jane's medium-term needs/problems. He has formulated a plan of care that addresses their needs in relation to the day of operation itself and has begun to complete the Theatre Checklist in conjunction with Bobby and Jane (Fig. 9.13).

References

1. Glasper, A., Stonehouse, J. & Martin, L. (1987) Core care plans. *Nursing Times*, **83** (10), 55–7.
2. Wright, S. (1987) Producing practical care plans. *Nursing Times*, **83** (10), 54.

CHILD'S HISTORY SHEET 2					

	Immunisation	Date or age administered:	Referrals made whilst in hospital, contact	Sign	Date
GP DR M SMALL Address ARNOLD HEALTH CENTRE FRONT STREET ARNOLD NG5 6PE Tel No. 267275	Dip] Tet] Polio Pert]	1st OCT '90 2nd NOV '90 3rd DEC '90			
Health Visitor NORA WRIGHT Address ARNOLD HEALTH CENTRE FRONT STREET ARNOLD NG5 6PE Tel No. 267275	Measles/Mumps/Rubella (YES)/NO Meningitis YES/NO Booster Dip. Tet. Polio (pre-school) YES/NO BCG Age administered N/A		Checklist for discharge info & referrals		
Health Centre Address AS ABOVE Tel No.	Booster Tet. & Polio School Leavers YES/NO Date of last Tetanus AS PER TRIPLE Reason immunisations not given:			Sign	Date
			Parent/child informed Discharge advice sheet given Equipment loaned		
Social Worker/other contacts OLIVE BLACK Other information SOCIAL WORKER'S TEL NO: 268932	Recent Contact with infectious diseases NONE KNOWN		Ward appt given to family OPD appt given to family Health Visitor informed Community Nurse informed Social Worker		
	Allergies ALLERGIC TO ELASTOPLAST		Doctor's Letter		

Ward Facilities - Tick box when explained to parents		Current medications & method of administration		Parent held records completed:	
Parents' Kitchen	✓	NOT ON ANY CURRENT MEDICINES		Yes	
Parents' Sitting/Smoking Room	✓	BUT WILL WILLINGLY TAKE LIQUID		No	
Ward Kitchen	✓	MEDICATIONS FROM A SPOON		N/A	
Parent information board/file	✓			Discharge weight	
Parent shower/toilet facilities	✓			Medications	
Telephone	✓				
Dining Room facilities	✓				
Family Care Assistant	✓	Signature of nurse taking history:	Date:		
Chaplaincy Department	✓	P. JONES	7|9|93		
Fire Regulations	✓	Signature of nurse checking:	Date:		
Facilities re-explained on ward transfer				Discharge Date	Time

Fig. 9.7 Case study 4: History Sheet 2.

CHILDREN'S UNIT – ASSESSMENT SHEET

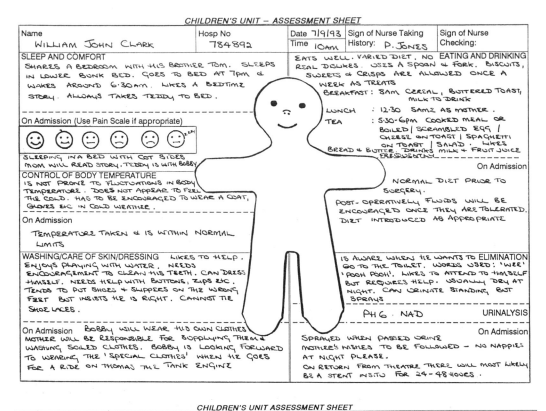

Name: WILLIAM JOHN CLARK	Hosp No 784892	Date 7/9/93 Time 10AM	Sign of Nurse Taking History: P. JONES	Sign of Nurse Checking:

SLEEP AND COMFORT
SHARES A BEDROOM WITH HIS BROTHER TOM. SLEEPS IN LOWER BUNK BED. GOES TO BED AT 7PM & WAKES AROUND 6.30AM. LIKES A BEDTIME STORY. ALWAYS TAKES TEDDY TO BED.

On Admission (Use Pain Scale if appropriate)

SLEEPING IN A BED WITH COT SIDES MOM WILL READ STORY. TEDDY IS WITH BOBBY

CONTROL OF BODY TEMPERATURE
IS NOT PRONE TO FLUCTUATIONS IN BODY TEMPERATURE. DOES NOT APPEAR TO FEEL THE COLD. HAS TO BE ENCOURAGED TO WEAR A COAT, GLOVES ETC IN COLD WEATHER.

On Admission
TEMPERATURE TAKEN & IS WITHIN NORMAL LIMITS

WASHING/CARE OF SKIN/DRESSING   LIKES TO HELP. ENJOYS PLAYING WITH WATER. NEEDS ENCOURAGEMENT TO CLEAN HIS TEETH. CAN DRESS HIMSELF. NEEDS HELP WITH BUTTONS, ZIPS ETC. TENDS TO PUT SHOES & SLIPPERS ON THE WRONG FEET BUT INSISTS HE IS RIGHT. CANNOT TIE SHOE LACES.

On Admission   BOBBY WILL WEAR HIS OWN CLOTHES MOTHER WILL BE RESPONSIBLE FOR SUPPLYING THEM & WASHING SOILED CLOTHES. BOBBY IS LOOKING FORWARD TO WEARING THE 'SPECIAL CLOTHES' WHEN HE GOES FOR A RIDE ON THOMAS THE TANK ENGINE

EATING AND DRINKING
EATS WELL. VARIED DIET. NO REAL DISLIKES. USES A SPOON & FORK. BISCUITS, SWEETS & CRISPS ARE ALLOWED ONCE A WEEK AS TREATS
BREAKFAST: 8AM CEREAL, BUTTERED TOAST, MILK TO DRINK
LUNCH   : 12.30 SAME AS MOTHER.
TEA   : 5.30-6PM COOKED MEAL OR BOILED / SCRAMBLED EGG / CHEESE ON TOAST / SPAGHETTI ON TOAST / SALAD. LIKES BREAD & BUTTER. DRINKS MILK & FRUIT JUICE FREQUENTLY.

On Admission
NORMAL DIET PRIOR TO SURGERY.
POST-OPERATIVELY FLUIDS WILL BE ENCOURAGED ONCE THEY ARE TOLERATED. DIET INTRODUCED AS APPROPRIATE

ELIMINATION
IS AWARE WHEN HE WANTS TO GO TO THE TOILET. WORDS USED: 'WEE' 'POOH POOH'. LIKES TO ATTEND TO HIMSELF BUT REQUIRES HELP. USUALLY DRY AT NIGHT. CAN URINATE STANDING BUT SPRAYS

PH 6. NAD   **URINALYSIS**

On Admission
SPRAYED WHEN PASSED URINE
MOTHER'S WISHES TO BE FOLLOWED – NO NAPPIES AT NIGHT PLEASE.
ON RETURN FROM THEATRE THERE WILL MOST LIKELY BE A STENT INSITU FOR 24-48 HOURS.

CHILDREN'S UNIT ASSESSMENT SHEET

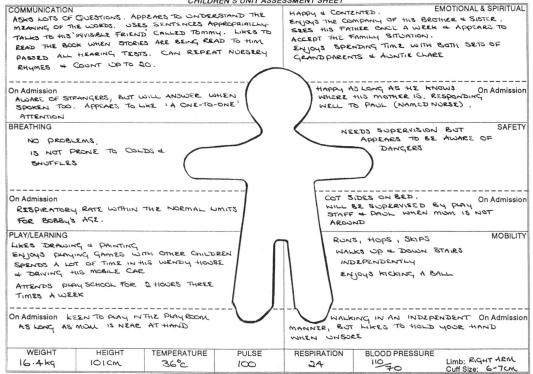

COMMUNICATION
ASKS LOTS OF QUESTIONS. APPEARS TO UNDERSTAND THE MEANING OF THE WORDS. USES SENTENCES APPROPRIATELY. TALKS TO HIS 'INVISIBLE FRIEND' CALLED TOMMY. LIKES TO READ THE BOOK WHEN STORIES ARE BEING READ TO HIM PASSED ALL HEARING TESTS. CAN REPEAT NURSERY RHYMES & COUNT UP TO 20.

On Admission
AWARE OF STRANGERS, BUT WILL ANSWER WHEN SPOKEN TOO. APPEARS TO LIKE 'A ONE-TO-ONE' ATTENTION

BREATHING
NO PROBLEMS.
IS NOT PRONE TO COLDS & SNUFFLES

On Admission
RESPIRATORY RATE WITHIN THE NORMAL LIMITS FOR BOBBY'S AGE.

PLAY/LEARNING
LIKES DRAWING & PAINTING
ENJOYS PLAYING GAMES WITH OTHER CHILDREN
SPENDS A LOT OF TIME IN HIS WENDY HOUSE & DRIVING HIS MOBILE CAR
ATTENDS PLAY SCHOOL FOR 2 HOURS THREE TIMES A WEEK

On Admission   KEEN TO PLAY IN THE PLAY ROOM AS LONG AS MOM IS NEAR AT HAND

EMOTIONAL & SPIRITUAL
HAPPY & CONTENTED.
ENJOYS THE COMPANY OF HIS BROTHER & SISTER. SEES HIS FATHER ONCE A WEEK & APPEARS TO ACCEPT THE FAMILY SITUATION.
ENJOYS SPENDING TIME WITH BOTH SETS OF GRANDPARENTS & AUNTIE CLARE

On Admission
HAPPY AS LONG AS HE KNOWS WHERE HIS MOTHER IS. RESPONDING WELL TO PAUL (NAMED NURSE).

SAFETY
NEEDS SUPERVISION BUT APPEARS TO BE AWARE OF DANGERS

On Admission
COT SIDES ON BED.
WILL BE SUPERVISED BY PLAY STAFF & PAUL WHEN MUM IS NOT AROUND

MOBILITY
RUNS, HOPS, SKIPS
WALKS UP & DOWN STAIRS INDEPENDENTLY
ENJOYS KICKING A BALL

On Admission
WALKING IN AN INDEPENDENT MANNER, BUT LIKES TO HOLD YOUR HAND WHEN UNSURE

WEIGHT	HEIGHT	TEMPERATURE	PULSE	RESPIRATION	BLOOD PRESSURE	
16.4 kg	101 cm	36°C	100	24	110/70	Limb: RIGHT ARM Cuff Size: 6-7 cm

Fig. 9.8 (facing page)
Case study 4: Assessment
Sheet (Gingerbread Man).

PAEDIATRIC NURSING CORE CARE PLAN					
PRE OPERATIVE AND PRE PROCEDURAL CARE (EMOTIONAL)					
NAME WILLIAM CLARK		HOSPITAL NO. 784892		AGE 3 YRS	
ACTIVITY OF LIVING .... EMOTIONAL			PROBLEM/NEED ....and family need clear explanations and support regarding the anaesthetic and procedure.		
DATE	TIME	NURSING ACTION PRE ANAESTHETIC CARE	AMEND ACTION Date Time & Sign	CHILD/PARENT ACTION	SIGN PARENT AND NURSE
7/9/93	9·30 AM	*Introduce self and other staff members to the child and family.	P. JONES 7/9/93 10AM		
		*Show around the ward areas and explain hospital facilities. SO THAT BOBBY & JANE BECOME FAMILIAR WITH THEIR ENVIRONMENT	P. JONES 7/9/93 10AM	JANE WILL SLEEP BY BOBBY'S BED & WILL USE WARD FACILITIES & RESTAURANT AT LUNCHTIME	J. CLARK
		*Explain all procedures to child and family. TO GIVE BOBBY & JANE APPROPRIATE KNOWLEDGE			
		*Answer any questions and queries to try and allay anxiety referring on to nurse in charge/doctor if appropriate.		BOBBY & JANE AWARE THEY CAN ASK QUESTIONS WHEN THEY SO WISH	J. CLARK
	11·30 AM	*Show appropriate video to help reduce stress if required. – PAUL TO ARRANGE	7/9/93 1200 P. JONES	BOBBY & JANE TO VIEW THE VIDEO	J. CLARK
8/9/93	8 AM	*Organise theatre clothing for carer to accompany child to theatre. SUE THEATRE NURSERY NURSE TO SHOW JANE HER THEATRE CLOTHING + TO BE AWARE OF TIME TO CHANGE + WHERE	7/9/93 1300 S. THORNHILL	JANE TO ACCOMPANY BOBBY TO THEATRE + TO STAY WITH HIM UNTIL HE GOES TO SLEEP. JANE WILL THEN CHANGE, HAVE BREAKFAST ON THE WARD & WAIT FOR BOBBY'S RETURN	J. CLARK.
					P. JONES.

Fig. 9.9 Case study 4: Nursing Core Care Plan – pre-anaesthetic and pre-procedural – emotional/spiritual.

<u>NURSING CARE PLAN – PROGRESS UPDATE</u>

NAME WILLIAM CLARK		HOSPITAL NO. 784892	AGE 3 YRS	
DATE	TIME	ACTIVITY OF LIVING EMOTIONAL ....PROBLEM/NEED NEED FOR CLEAR EXPLANATION RE: ANAESTHETIC & PROCEDURE		SIGN
7/9/93	9 30 AM	BOBBY & JANE INTRODUCED TO OTHER MEMBERS OF STAFF & SHOWN AROUND THE WARD		P. JONES
	12.00	BOBBY & JANE HAVE SEEN THE VIDEO. JANE REQUESTED INDEPTH INFORMATION REGARDING ANAESTHETIC & OPERATIVE PROCEDURES. EXPLANATION, INFORMATION & REASSURANCE GIVEN. TO BE SEEN BY DOCTOR & ANAESTHETIST LATER TODAY		P. JONES
	13.00	JANE SHOWN THEATRE CLOTHING & KNOWS WHAT TIME TO CHANGE & WHERE		S. THORNHILL

Fig. 9.10 Case study 4: Progress Update – emotional/spiritual.

PAEDIATRIC NURSING CORE CARE PLAN					
PRE ANAESTHETIC CARE (SAFETY)					

NAME ....WILLIAM CLARK......   HOSPITAL NO. ...784892.......   AGE ...3YRS..........

ACTIVITY OF LIVING ....SAFETY .... PROBLEM/NEED ...BOBBY...is having a general anaesthetic and needs
to be safely cared for pre-anaesthetic

DATE	TIME	NURSING ACTION PRE ANAESTHETIC CARE	AMEND ACTION Date Time & Sign	CHILD/PARENT ACTION	SIGN PARENT AND NURSE
7/9/93	9.30am	* Record base line observation of temp, pulse, respiratory rate and blood pressure.	7/9/93 10AM P. JONES		
		Report any abnormality to nurse in charge/doctor.			
		REPEAT BOBBY'S TPR AT 8AM ON 8/9/93			
		* Ensure that pre-medication has been prescribed to avoid delay.			
		* Ensure that cots sides are in situ to prevent falls.	7/9/93 10AM P. JONES		
		* Record the time the doctor informed of arrival to avoid confusion.	7/9/93 11 AM P. JONES		
		* Ensure oxygen and suction are available and in working order, near to the bedside.	7/9/93 10AM P. JONES		
		RE-CHECK AT 8AM ON 8/9/93			
		* Complete theatre checklist.			
8/9/93	08.00	* Nil by mouth from .....08.00..............			
		BOBBY CAN HAVE CLEAR FLUIDS (FRUIT JUICE) UP TO 3 HOURS PRIOR TO SURGERY – BOBBY WILL BE GOING TO THEATRE AT 11AM ON 8/9/93		JANE WILL GIVE BOBBY HIS LAST DRINK AT 8AM ON 8/9/93 & TAKE HIM FOR A WALK WHILST THE OTHER CHILDREN HAVE BREAKFAST	J. CLARK.
7/9/93	10AM	IDENTITY BRACELET COMPLETED & ATTACHED TO BOBBY'S RIGHT WRIST	7/9/93 10AM P. JONES		
					P. JONES

CHILDREN'S UNIT PRE–OPERATIVE THEATRE CHECKLIST

AFFIX BAR CODE LABEL

	CHECKLIST	WARD CIRCLE			THEATRE CIRCLE			CHECKLIST	WARD CIRCLE	
		N/A	Y	N	N/A	Y	N	Completed notes	Y	N
	Operation Gown & bath	N/A	Y	N	N/A	Y	N			
	Jewellery removed	(N/A)	Y	N	N/A	Y	N	X–rays	(N/A) Y	N
	Make–up/nail varnish removed	(N/A)	Y	N	N/A	Y	N	Sickle Cell result	(N/A) Y	N
Date: 7/9/93 Time: 11-00								Child/parents prepared for High Dependency area	(N/A) Y	N
Child's Name: WILLIAM CLARK Address: 29 RUSHWOOD CRESENT ARNOLD	Prothesis/contact lenses removed	(N/A)	Y	N	N/A	Y	N	Parent & Nurse to accompany child	(Y)	N
Hospital No: 784892	Braces removed	(N/A)	Y	N	N/A	Y	N	Toy/comforter accompanying	(Y)	N
Ward: CEDAR	Loose teeth	N/A	Y	(N)	N/A	Y	N	Removed sutures etc, wanted		
Consultant: MR SCOTT	Capped crowned teeth	(N/A)	Y	N	N/A	Y	N	by child	(N/A) Y	N
Proposed Operation: REPAIR OF GLANDULAR HYPOSPADIAS	Identification bracelet checked	N/A	Y	N	N/A	Y	N	Explanation of procedure to: Child	Y	N
	Allergy band	N/A	Y	N	N/A	Y	N	Carer	Y	N
Allergies: (write in red) ELASTOPLAST	Consent signed		Y	N		Y	N	Any phobia/anxiety	Y	N
	Pre–medication given	N/A	Y	N	N/A	Y	N			
	Topical precannulation cream	N/A	Y	N	N/A	Y	N			
Special needs relevant to theatre care:	Theatre tag checked	N/A	Y	N	N/A	Y	N			
	Fasted from: Diet Fluids	Time						Special instruction/preparation	Y	N
Pre–operative Observations T P R BP Cuff Size Limb 36°c 100 24 110/70 RIGHT ARM	KEY: N/A = Not Applicable Y = YES N = NO									
Weight Urinalysis 16.4kg PH6 NAD	Theatre Nurse Signature: Date: Time:							Ward Nurse Signature: Date: Time:		

Fig. 9.11 (facing page top) Case study 4: Nursing Core Care Plan – pre-anaesthetic – safety.

NURSING CARE PLAN – PROGRESS UPDATE

NAME WILLIAM CLARK		HOSPITAL NO 784.892	AGE 3 YES

DATE	TIME	ACTIVITY OF LIVING SAFETY PROBLEM/NEED BOBBY IS HAVING A GENERAL ANAESTHETIC & NEEDS TO BE SAFELY CARED FOR PRE-ANAESTHETIC SIGN	
7/9/93	10 AM	BASELINE OBSERVATIONS OF TEMPERATURE, PULSE, RESPIRATORY RATE & BLOOD PRESSURE WITHIN NORMAL LIMITS	P. JONES
	11 AM	BASELINE OBSERVATIONS RECORDED ON THEATRE CHECKLIST. DOCTOR INFORMED OF BOBBY'S ARRIVAL	P. JONES

Fig. 9.12 Case study 4: Progress Update – safety.

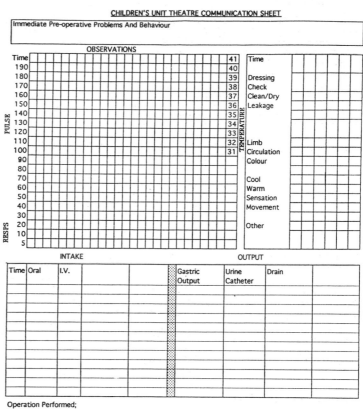

Fig. 9.13 (facing page bottom and right) Case study 4: Theatre Checklist (partially completed).

Part 4

From Hospital to Home

Chapter 10
Facilitating Care at Home

Over recent years there has been a growing emphasis towards community and preventive health care. Numerous reports, such as *Community Care: Agenda For Action* [1], as well as the Department of Health document *Caring For People* [2], reinforce the ideal that patients should be cared for in their own homes whenever possible. As far back as 1955 the World Health Organization stated that:

'The best place to care for a sick child is in his own home among familiar surroundings where the people who normally give him security and affection can tend to his needs' [3].

This was reiterrated by the Platt Report [4] which stressed that children should be treated at home by their GP whenever possible and that hospital admissions should be avoided unless absolutely necessary. The Court Report [5] also advocated care at home and stressed that, 'The importance of the family must be reflected in the organization and delivery of health services for children.'

In recognition of the fact that the best place for sick children to be cared for is in their own homes, by their families, a number of children's units over recent years have developed paediatric community nursing teams to not only aid the transition from hospital to home, but also to offer an alternative to hospital-based care. However, the Audit Commission in 1986 [6] highlighted that developments in this area have been somewhat patchy, with the result being that for many children and families their need for such a service continues to be unmet.

The need to increase the availability of paediatric community nursing teams is therefore seen as extremely important. The Department of Health document *Welfare of Children and Young People in Hospital* [7] states that:

'Where they exist, paediatric community nursing services can make a very helpful contribution to the support of families caring for sick children at home.'

Indeed, the document [7] stresses:

- Their value in achieving continuity of health care.
- Their role in facilitating earlier discharges.
- Their role in the prevention of hospital admissions.

- Their role in reducing the visits to hospital for post-operative wound checks or investigations such as blood tests.

Belson [8] and others [9–10] highlight the fact that up to 25–30 per cent of admissions could be prevented by the provision of such a service. Others [10–16] also clearly highlight that the length of hospital stays can be reduced quite considerably if there are appropriately skilled nurses to provide care and support for families at home. The Audit Commission [17] indicates that although the number of children admitted to hospital has increased over recent years, the average length of stay has fallen. This is seen to be due to:

- An increase in day surgery.
- The involvement of parents at an earlier stage within their child's care in hospital, thereby increasing their confidence and competence to perform care at home.
- An increase in the provision of community services by RSCNs, thereby facilitating the provision of specialist care at home.

In particular, the latter is attributed to:

- An increase in the demand for home-based care from parents and families.
- Improved technology enabling procedures to be undertaken at home.
- Increased awareness that home-based care yields the same level of outcome and is more cost-effective than care in hospital [18–19].

An alternative to hospital-based care

There is a wealth of research that demonstrates and clearly highlights the detrimental and far-reaching psychological effects that a period of hospitalization can have upon a young child [20–26]. The root cause of emotional disturbance amongst children is seen to be the direct result of separation from their parents and family, as well as from their normal environment. Although most children's units now offer facilities for parents and other family members to remain with their child, many are unable to do so for a variety of reasons.

Couriel *et al.* [27] indicate that parents with other children experience a great deal of conflict over their desire to be with the sick child and the guilt if they do so, as they feel they are neglecting the needs of their other children. Other factors such as work commitments or a fear of the hospital environment may mean that they may be unwilling to stay [28]. There are also numerous financial implications associated with a period of hospitalization. Costs include travelling expenses, child care provision for siblings and the cost of food as a resident parent.

The provision of a service that facilitates home care avoids not only the detrimental effects of hospitalization, as the child is cared for by his/her usual carers in familiar surroundings, but also additional costs to the family. The benefits of such a service are shown in Table 10.1. In this respect, there are also benefits of preserving the integrity of the family unit for other siblings, as well as for the sick child. Facilitating care at home also enables the child and family to lead a more normal lifestyle, as well as to retain their independence and control over the situation.

Table 10.1 The benefits of a paediatric community nursing service.

- Facilitates shorter hospital stays.
- Reduces effects of hospitalization and separation from the family.
- Reduces the risk of cross-infection.
- Reduces the disruption to the family unit and their lifestyle.
- Decreases the time and expense involved in visiting the hospital or being resident in hospital.
- Provides the opportunity for health education at home.
- Gives continuity in care.
- Reduces health service costs.
- Reduces the number of hospital attendances, e.g. ward attenders/out-patient assessments.
- Provides support for families providing care at home.
- Reduces the time children are absent from school and their usual activities.

There are numerous studies that indicate that parents are capable of performing quite complex tasks, providing they have been given the opportunity to learn the techniques [8, 29–32]. Care provided at home by parents can range from gastrostomy or naso-gastric tube feeds, to the administration of intravenous medication, tracheostomy care and peritoneal dialysis, as well as caring for the child who is terminally ill who requires the administration of pain relief.

However, Martin [33] highlights that many parents experience a great deal of stress related to the responsibility of providing treatment at home. The provision of support, advice and encouragement are therefore seen as vital elements of the paediatric community nurse's role. Factors such as access to specialist advice, as well as an 'open door' policy enabling the child to return to hospital at any time, have been found to influence the parent's decision to care for their child at home [34–37].

While [9] states that most parents view the possibility of providing care at home as an acceptable and welcome alternative to hospital-based care, but Martin [33] indicates that for some the obligation for a parent to remain at home may also present problems where both parents work. Dufour [37] and Martinson *et al.* [38], however, indicate that it is imperative that parents are given the opportunity to care for their child at home whenever possible. This is particularly important when the child is dying, as facilitating and supporting the family to provide care at home assists with their adaptation and acceptance following the child's death.

Fradd [39] states that the provision of a service that enables a sick child to be cared for at home:

'. . . brings together all the important philosophical thoughts that pae-diatric nurses believe in, such as parental involvement, an appropriate environment, choice and "what is in the best interests of the child".'

In the past, many parents would not have been given the opportunity to care for their child at home if they required complex or technical care. Yet, today, with the recognition that the best place for a sick child to be cared for is in their own home, by their family, many are now supported in doing so by appropriately skilled nurses.

The role of the paediatric community nurse

Figure 10.1 highlights the key role of the paediatric community nurse as the link between the child and family, the hospital staff and the primary health care team. The involvement of a paediatric community nurse is seen to facilitate better communication between the hospital and the primary health care team, with the result that care is better co-ordinated and appropriately geared towards the needs of each individual child and family [8, 13–14, 40].

In addition, a recent publication by the Royal College of Nursing [41] concerning paediatric community nurses, lists the following regarding the contribution they can make to the care of ill children and their families:

- Assess the particular needs of a family that has a sick child within it.
- Enable children to be nursed in community settings, for example, playgroup, nurseries, residential homes, respite care facilities and their own homes.
- Enable children with a debilitating disease to fulfil their potential, enhancing their quality of life.
- Provide opportunistic health promotion for the whole family.
- Plan, in co-operation with the family, the special nursing needs of the ill child.
- At the end of life, enable the child to die with dignity in the place of his/ her choice.
- Provide crisis intervention, thus offering continual support to families who live with a high level of stress associated with caring for a child with a chronic illness.
- Enable parents to feel confident and competent when caring for their child.
- Teach families to carry out specific nursing care, including high-tech procedures.
- Act as an interface between community, hospital and all other agen-cies, for example, cubs, school camps or sports camps, providing continuity of care and facilitating the normal activities of childhood and adolescence.
- Help families network with others, reducing feelings of isolation and despair.

Fig. 10.1 The role of the paediatric community nurse.

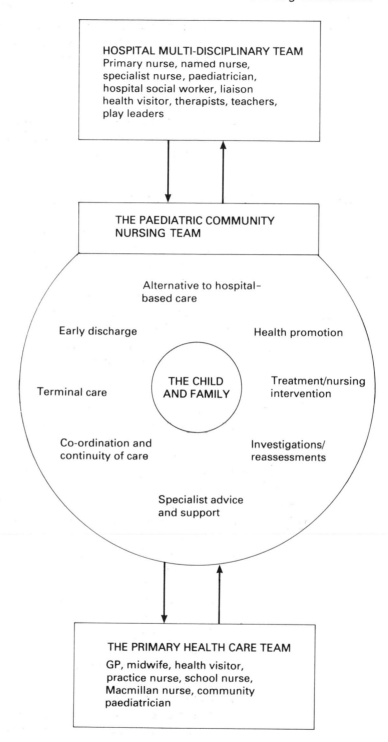

HOSPITAL MULTI-DISCIPLINARY TEAM
Primary nurse, named nurse, specialist nurse, paediatrician, hospital social worker, liaison health visitor, therapists, teachers, play leaders

THE PAEDIATRIC COMMUNITY NURSING TEAM

Alternative to hospital–based care

Early discharge

Health promotion

Terminal care

THE CHILD AND FAMILY

Treatment/nursing intervention

Co-ordination and continuity of care

Investigations/ reassessments

Specialist advice and support

THE PRIMARY HEALTH CARE TEAM

GP, midwife, health visitor, practice nurse, school nurse, Macmillan nurse, community paediatrician

- Offer appropriate support and help following bereavement.
- Prevent hospital admission and attendance. Paediatric community nurses can also facilitate early discharge while the option of day care is made more readily available.
- Teach student nurses, community nurses, medical students, GP trainees and others.
- Act as a specialist resource for all health care workers.
- In common with district nurses and health visitors, paediatric community nurses will be able to prescribe certain medicines once the regulations are in place.

Maintaining continuity in the approach to care

The philosophy of the Children's Unit in Nottingham [see chapter 2] reflects the view that the best place for a sick child to be cared for is in his/her own home, by his/her family. Children are therefore nursed at home whenever possible and/or discharged home at the earliest conceivable time. In order to achieve this goal, an effective and appropriately skilled community nursing team has developed to support the family in delivering care at home. The provision of a paediatric community nursing service enables children to be discharged home much earlier and in some instances prevents that initial admission to hospital.

The philosophy is to maintain the integrity of the family unit, promote care by the family and enable the family to maintain its independence. This approach also recognizes the importance of family relationships and other social factors which are relevant to the individual child. The emphasis is upon teaching the parents and the family, health education and the provision of long-term support, guidance and advice, as well as specialist nursing intervention.

Preparation for discharge begins on admission, at which time the named nurse or primary nurse assesses the child and family's needs and plans their immediate and long-term care. Essentially, it is this nurse's responsibility to:

- make the initial contact with the community nurse well in advance of a child's potential discharge; and
- then continue to liaise with and assist in preparing the child and family for continuing treatment or care at home.

During this pre-discharge period, the community nurse meets frequently with the child, parents and family on the ward. This enables the nurse to not only develop a friendship and form an allegiance, but also to become the key figure in the process that is involved in preparing for the continuation of treatment or care at home.

The philosophy of the Children's Unit recognizes the importance of maintaining continuity in the child and family's care, whether this is by a named nurse, primary nurse, specialist or community nurse. The model itself centres around a child and family focused approach and parental participation in care giving, whether in the hospital or at home. In order to achieve these goals it is imperative that there is harmony in the approach to care, between the hospital and the home, a fact that is recognized and encompassed within this model of care.

In order to attain this co-ordinated approach to care and continuity, the same procedures and protocols are followed whether the child is in hospital or at home, or whether carried out by the nurse or the family. However, in recognition of the different environment and the altered needs of the child and family, the community nursing team utilize an adapted version of the Gingerbread Man Assessment Sheet (Fig. 10.2), as well as a Community Referral and History Sheet 1 and 2 (Fig. 10.3). The Community Referral and History Sheet 1 and 2 forms the basis of information regarding the child and family's initial care requirements following discharge home.

Care plans and other records require adaptation to reflect different environments and circumstances. However, the use of nursing records between hospital and home and vice versa promotes good communication between professionals, the child and family, and also assists in the maintenance of a unified approach to caring.

The community nursing records

The nursing records remain in the home throughout the duration of the child's care. This facilitates:

- a child and family focused approach;
- child and family participation; and
- the recording and evaluation of care.

The community nursing team use the same nursing records as those used by hospital-based nurses. These are presented in Part 2 and the same guidelines apply. However, a specifically designed Community Referral and History Sheet 1 and 2 (see Fig. 10.3) replaces the History Sheet(s) 1 and 2 (Figs. 3.1 and 3.2) utilized within the hospital, and provides the link between hospital and home-based care. In addition, the Gingerbread Man Assessment Sheet has been slightly altered (Fig. 10.2).

All children referred to the community nursing team must have the Community Referral and History Sheet(s) 1 and 2 (Fig. 10.3) completed prior to acceptance by the community nursing team. These nursing records are divided into two main sections:

- Section 1: to be completed by the child's and family's primary nurse or named nurse.
- Section 2: to be completed by the child's and family's community nurse during the first home visit.

Early completion and referral by the primary or named nurse is desirable in

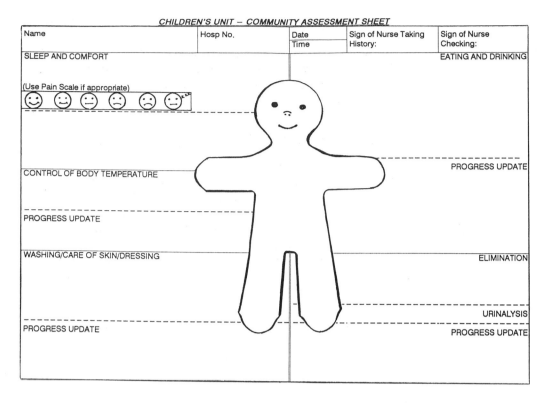

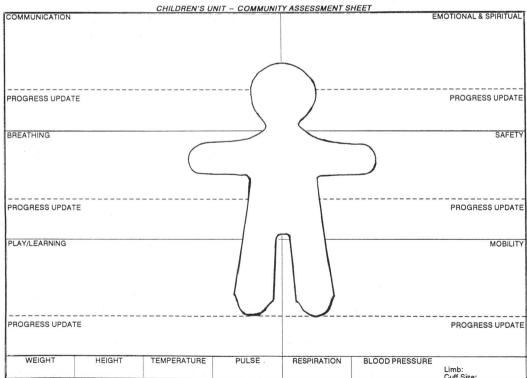

Fig. 10.2 (facing page)
Community Assessment
(Gingerbread Man) Sheet.

order to facilitate discharge and the continuation of care/treatment at home.

The Community Referral and History Sheet(s) 1 and 2 are collected from the wards by the community nursing team, who are responsible for ensuring that the Community Referral and History Sheet(s) 1 and 2 are completed correctly.

Guidelines for the Community Referral and History Sheet 1

This must be completed by the primary nurse or named nurse, and as with all nursing records it must be signed and dated in the relevant areas. The required information is obtained from the child's nursing records and checked with the child (depending upon his/her age, maturity, cognitive level and ability) and his/her parents or carers.

For guidelines on personal details, time, date and reason for admission and referrals made whilst in hospital, refer to *History Sheet Guidelines*, chapter 3.

What information have parents been given about diagnosis/ condition of their child?

Include details related to diagnosis and the outcome of investigations, prognosis and the long-term management of the child's treatment/care.

Nursing needs on discharge

Any specific nursing care required, e.g. naso-gastric tube feeding, wound care, the administration of intravenous antibiotics, tracheostomy care, etc.

Supplies needed

Any equipment or type of dressing, wound care products, etc. required to meet the child's nursing needs.

Guidelines for the Community Referral and History Sheet 2

Other information

Used to note any other information that may be relevant to the child's care at home, e.g. previous referral to the community nursing team, the time of day that the parent or child may not be at their home address.

Medication

Details of all medications, including (where possible) dosage, frequency and method of administration should be recorded in this section.

Nursing procedures taught to and undertaken by carers/child

All procedures that the parents/carers and child have been taught and are competent and confident to perform at home, e.g. bolus naso-gastric

Section One: To be completed by Ward Nurse	CHILD'S COMMUNITY REFERRAL AND HISTORY SHEET 1	REG NO:
WARD:		
Family Name:	Date: Time:	Nursery/School:
First Name:	Reason for referral to Community Team	
Likes to be called:		Names and ages of siblings:
Age:		
DOB:		
Birth weight:	Medical Diagnosis:	
Religion: Christened: YES/NO		Nursing needs on discharge:
Child's Address:	Reason for admission to hospital	
Postcode:		
Telephone No:		
Next of Kin: Relationship to child: Address if different from above:		Supplies needed:
	GP: Address:	
	Tel No:	
Telephone No: Work: Home:	Health Visitor: Address:	
With whom does the child reside:		Referrals made whilst in hospital :
	Tel No:	Contact name	Tel No	Title	Date
Like to be called: Relationship to Child:	Health Centre: Address:	
Who has parental responsibility for this child?:		
	Tel No:	
Telephone number:	Social Worker/other contacts:	
Child's Ward Nurse/Team:	Consultant:	

To be completed by Ward Nurse		Section Two: To be completed by Community Sister	
Appointment given: Date: Time: OPD/Ward: Allergies:	Nursing procedures taught to and undertaken by carers/child:	Why do the parents think the child is being visited:	Equipment - Serial Numbers (tick if Disclaimer Form signed)
		What reason does the child give for being visited (if applicable):	
Other Information:			Other relevant information:
		Social Arrangements:	
	Procedures not being undertaken by carers/child:		
Current medications & method of administration:			
		History taken from: (relationship to child)	
	Signature of Nurse referring: Date:	Signature of Community Nurse taking history Date:	Child's Community Named Nurse
Discharge Date & Time:			

Fig. 10.3 (facing page)
Community Referral and
History Sheet 1 and 2.

feeding, passing a naso-gastric tube, flushing a Hickman line, redressing a wound, etc.

Procedures not being undertaken by carers/child

Procedures that the parents/carers and child do not wish to or are not competent or confident to perform at home. All the procedures a child requires should be noted in one or other of the above sections.

Social arrangements

Details recorded should be brief and informative, e.g. transport needs or difficulties, additional assistance required by the family to enable them to care for the child at home, family support network/responsibilities. Subjective and judgemental comments should *not* be made.

Other relevant information

Once the Community Referral and History Sheet 2 have been completed, the community nurse must ascertain from the parents/carers if there is any other information that may affect the child's care/treatment at home, e.g. mother is pregnant, father works away from home, another sibling is unwell with flu, etc. This section is also used to communicate any important information about the child and family to other members of the community nursing team. Therefore the information may duplicate that contained elsewhere on the Community Referral and History Sheet(s) 1 and 2.

Guidelines for the Community Assessment Sheet – 'Gingerbread Man'

The Assessment Sheet (Fig. 10.2) has been adapted for use in the community. Its aim is to:

- Gain a comprehensive outline of the child's usual routine.
- Identify the Activities of Living that have altered due to the child's present condition or illness.
- Identify the child and family's perception of progress made since hospital admission and/or the commencement of treatment.

The guidelines outlined in chapter 3 are applicable to the section pertaining to the child's usual routine and Activities of Living.

The 'Progress Update' section

The child's Activities of Living may differ from his/her usual Activities of Living. It is these differences that should be recorded in this section, along with information regarding the child and family's perception, and the community nurse's assessment, of progress made since admission and/or commencement of treatment. If any of the child's Activities of Living are unchanged from his/her usual, 'No change' should be written in the appropriate section, along with a statement reflecting the child's present health state.

The Children's Clinic: the final link in the continuum of care

Many professionals, as a result of misconceptions and preconceived ideas, fail to fully acknowledge or recognize the valuable role that out-patient services play in enabling children to be cared for in the community. Often they are perceived as low priority areas, with resources being directed elsewhere [42]. However, the Platt Report [4] states that:

> 'Children should only be admitted to hospital when the medical treatment they require cannot be given in other ways without real disadvantage.'

Attendance at appropriate and accessible out-patient clinics, where advice, care or treatment can be given, can therefore be seen as one of the means to facilitate a child's parents and family to care for the child at home, thereby preventing the emotional trauma associated with a period of hospitalization.

The Department of Health document *Welfare of Children and Young People in Hospital* [7] reinforces this fact by stating that:

> 'Children should only be admitted to hospital if the care they require cannot be ... provided at home, in a day clinic or on a day basis in hospital.'

In recognition of the fact that for many children their first encounter of a hospital is at an out-patient clinic, the document [7] recommends:

- The provision of facilities that are appropriately geared towards meeting the needs of children and their families.
- A service that also reflects the philosophy of the Children's Unit, including continuity in the approach to caring and parental participation in the delivery of care.

The important role and function of the Children's Clinic should be perceived as the final link in the continuum of the caring process. It must, however, be noted that for many children the Children's Clinic or Out-patient Department may be the first or only contact with secondary care. Therefore, for these children the Children's Clinic may be perceived as the first link.

Whilst attending the clinic for review by paediatricians, the child and family may also be seen by a wide range of other specialists, including clinical psychologists, speech therapists or by one of the many specialist nurses, for example, the asthma, cystic fibrosis, diabetic, renal, family therapy or oncology specialist nurses. They provide the link between the ward and the clinic. Their role is to assess and plan care in respect of the child's and family's special needs whether on the ward, in the clinic or at home. The ultimate goal, however, is to enable the child's primary nurse to be present during such clinic attendances, in order that they can continue to assess needs, plan care and provide continued support to the child and family. This may occur occasionally, but due to organizational difficulties it is not always feasible. Instead, many children and families visit the ward following attendance at clinics in order to see their primary or special nurse. It should be noted that staff within the Out-patient Department may act as the child and family's named or primary nurse if the child has not previously been an in-patient.

Children with chronic illnesses or progressive diseases spend a large proportion of their lives in hospital, attending clinics and being cared for at home by their family. It is therefore essential that a harmonized approach to care is maintained, whether the child is nursed at home or in hospital, by a named nurse, primary nurse, specialist or community nurse. Figure 10.4 indicates the significance of each of these nurses in the continuum of care. The importance of good communication and co-operation between all concerned in caring for an individual child and his/her family cannot be overstated.

Fig. 10.4 The continuum of nursing care: hospital to home.

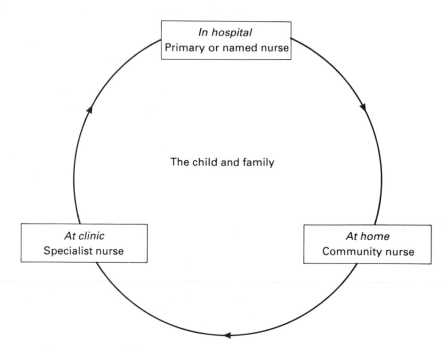

Case study 5
Jo Williamson: enabling care to continue at home

The following case study demonstrates the application of the Nottingham model and the associated nursing records within the community. It also highlights:

- The use of a referral sheet, providing the link between hospital and home-based care.
- The adaptation of the Gingerbread Man to facilitate the recording of different information.

- Shared care between hospital-based and community-based professionals, as well as the child and family.
- The valuable role of a link nurse and community nurse, as well as a multi-disciplinary approach to the care of a child with a chronic illness. The latter facilitates the provision of the optimum level of care to meet the child's needs and those of the family.
- The use of shared procedures and protocols between the hospital and community.
- The value of providing specific education and training geared towards children and their families, thereby enabling them to attain the knowledge and acquire the skills to competently perform care at home.

Jo Williamson is an eight-year-old girl with cystic fibrosis. Cystic fibrosis (CF) is the commonest genetic disease affecting Caucasians. One in twenty of the population in the UK carry the gene that is responsible for CF. Where both parents carry this gene they have a 1:4 chance of having an affected child. Children with CF usually present with symptoms during early infancy, and have respiratory as well as digestive problems. Treatment includes twice daily physiotherapy, prompt treatment of chest infections and, in order to aid the absorption of food, the consumption of pancreatic enzymes.

Although prognosis and longevity has improved with better management, there is still no known cure. Caring for a child with a chronic illness, performing daily treatment and the effect of recurrent chest infections which often necessitate frequent admission to hospital, have a considerable impact upon the life of the child and his/her family.

Over the last year Jo has had repeated chest infections for which she has required admission for intravenous antibiotics and intensive physiotherapy. The admission to Beaver ward was Jo's third admission within a 12-month period.

On a previous admission Jo's parents expressed a desire to continue her care at home whenever possible. Jo and her parents therefore attended a study evening to learn the techniques and safety aspects involved in the administration of intravenous therapy. Table 10.2 outlines the content of the study evening that Jo and her parents attended. On the last admission Jo and her parents completed a practical teaching programme on the ward and were assessed by the cystic fibrosis link nurse as being competent to perform this procedure according to the Children's Unit policy and procedure. In addition to the latter, children and families undertaking the administration of intravenous drugs are also provided with guidelines and an *aide-mémoire* (Tables 10.3 and 10.4).

On admission Clare Welch (Jo's primary nurse) identified that Jo and her parents felt confident to continue the administration of intravenous antibiotics at home via her infusion device (Table 10.5 and Fig. 10.5). Whilst the nursing records relating to the duration of Jo's stay on Beaver ward have not been included in this book, discharge planning began at the point of admission. The care plans that were formulated by Clare addressed the issues relating to preparing for Jo's discharge. They included:

- Re-assessing both Jo's and her parents' knowledge and competence in the administration of intravenous antibiotics.
- Reinforcing the need for increased physiotherapy during the course of treatment.

Table 10.2 A study evening to prepare chiildren and families for home intravenous (IV) therapy.

Formal training in aspects of home IV care for children with cystic fibrosis has developed to meet an increasing need. Children and families who choose to learn the techniques and safety aspects involved are invited to attend an IV study evening prior to the commencement of a practical teaching programme on the ward. The study sessions are held during the evening so as not to disrupt work or school life. This thereby enables all family members who may be involved with the child's care to attend, including grandparents, brothers and sisters.

The study evening centres around a team approach and involves the cystic fibrosis link nurse, infection control sister, paediatric community nurse, a pharmacist and the community physiotherapist. The main aim is to prepare the child and family by giving them all the basic information they require before being taught how to administer the drugs themselves. The content of the evening includes:

- The advantages and disadvantages of home IV therapy.
- The commonly used drugs and their side effects.
- The possible complications and risks involved and what to do if problems occur.
- Familiarization with the equipment used in the administration of IV therapy at home.
- Safe hand-washing and storage/preparation of drugs.
- Why more frequent physiotherapy is essential during the course of IV treatment.

Once the study evening has been attended, practical teaching begins on the next admission at which time an individual care plan is negotiated to address the practical teaching and training required. Theoretical teaching is reinforced by a specifically designed workbook which must be completed before a Certificate of Competence* can be awarded. Competency must be achieved before children are allowed to be discharged home on IV medication.

* It should be noted that the Children's Unit is moving towards the use of 'A Record of Teaching for Parents/Families' rather than the use of Certificates of Competence.

The completed Community Referral and History Sheet 1 (Fig. 10.6) indicates that preparation for discharge included contacting:

- Sarah Blunt (the hospital physiotherapist).
- John Olds (the hospital school teacher).
- June Brown (the dietician).
- Ann Winters (the paediatric community nurse).
- Helen Downs (the CF specialist social worker).
- Sheila Dent (the Community physiotherapist).

The early involvement of those mentioned above thereby ensured that all the necessary arrangements were made by the multi-disciplinary team in order to facilitate Jo's discharge. Although Ann Winters was already known to Jo and her

Table 10.3 Guidelines for children and families regarding home intravenous drug therapy (utilized in conjunction with the Children's Unit IV drug therapy policies and procedures).

(1) The intravenous drug therapy study evening must be attended before a child/family can give intravenous drugs at home unsupervised.

(2) The child/family will have a period of training in the giving of intravenous drugs during a ward admission. This training will be negotiated with the family and documented in the care plan. The child/family should be observed drawing up and giving drugs at least five times using a safe technique by a trained member of staff who holds the Nottingham Health Authority Certificate of Competence for giving intravenous medication to children.

(3) Following the education programme, a child/family should be able to do the following before discharge:

- Demonstrate how to administer intravenous drugs safely and competently.
- Name the drugs being used and the reasons for taking them.
- State dosages and the timings of the drugs to be given.
- Name possible (common) side effects of the drugs.
- State the possible complications that may be encountered when giving intravenous drugs.
- Demonstrate a knowledge of safety aspects including hand-washing, disposal of sharps and equipment, and drug reaction.
- Keep an accurate record of the medication administered on the drug/medication sheet.

(4) Children/families should be aware of the intravenous drug policies and procedures applicable to the Children's Unit. Copies of the relevant policies should be given to them.

(5) An intravenous therapy certificate will be completed for each family member/child who has been assessed as competent to give intravenous drugs at home.

(6) The first dose of the drug course will always be given in hospital by a member of the medical staff to allow observation for drug reactions.

(7) The family will be discharged home following full consultation with them, at the discretion of nursing and medical staff. Adequate support in the community should be assured before discharge.

(8) Those children going home on the home intravenous drug delivery system must give the manufacturing company 48 hours' notice by fax (see procedure for sending a patient home on the home intravenous antibiotic system).

(9) The child/family must be given contact numbers for those involved in community support.

(10) A loan form must be completed if the family are to take any hospital equipment home in order to administer intravenous drugs. The relevance of the form must be explained to them.

(11) The family must be given the drug prescription and administration record from the ward, signed by the medical staff, to enable them to keep an accurate record of medications administered at home, and to enable them to check the drugs and doses against the prescription before they are administered.

Table 10.3 *Continued*

---

(12) The child/family should be given all relevant information sheets from the ward before discharge.

(13) All drugs and equipment to be taken home must be checked by a trained member of staff to ensure the family have all the correct supplies on discharge and that they understand how to administer them.

(14) The family must be aware of immediately reporting any problems encountered when at home to the paediatric community nurse or the ward team.

(15) All families will be contacted or visited within 72 hours of going home and will receive at least one other visit from the paediatric community nurse during the course of intravenous therapy. This will allow continual assessment of skills and updating of knowledge and ensure that any problems encountered are managed as quickly as possible.

(16) Weight and vitalograph readings will be recorded and sputum specimens collected at the beginning, middle and end of the course of home intravenous antibiotic therapy. This must be recorded on a home assessment sheet and a copy of this placed in the medical and nursing notes.

(17) Blood samples for tobramycin and gentamicin levels can be collected at home using 'finger prick' on the request of medical staff.

(18) Extra physiotherapy must be given by the family during a course of home intravenous antibiotic therapy. The community physiotherapist will assess the need for physiotherapy and may visit the child and family at home.

(19) When the last dose of antibiotics has been administered at home, the long line can be removed by the paediatric community nurse.

(20) An out-patient clinic appointment must be made for no more than four weeks after the end of the course of home intravenous therapy.

---

family (as she was present at the study evening regarding Home Intravenous Therapy which they attended), Clare contacted her and arranged for Ann to meet with Jo and her parents whilst Jo was still an in-patient on Beaver ward. This provided Ann with the opportunity to gain an insight into the needs of the family and to become a key member in the process of preparing for treatment to continue at home.

The completed Community Referral and History Sheet(s) 1 and 2 (Fig. 10.6) indicate:

● Jo's nursing needs on discharge.
● The supplies required.
● The nursing procedures taught to and being undertaken by Jo and her parents.
● Those procedures that the paediatric community nurse will be required to perform during Jo's period of intravenous antibiotic treatment at home.

The names, telephone numbers and addresses of all those individuals involved in Jo's care can also be found on the Community Referral and History Sheet 1 (Fig. 10.6). This highlights the involvement of numerous professionals within the care and treatment of a child with a chronic illness, and includes details of all the

Table 10.4 An aide-mémoire for children and families: the giving of intravenous drugs (utilized in conjunction with the Children's Unit IV drug therapy policies and procedures).

(1) All drugs should be stored at room temperature, preferably in a cupboard.
(2) Find a clear surface for getting drugs ready.
(3) Make sure the surface is cleaned before use.
(4) Get out all the equipment needed.
(5) Wash hands.
(6) Intravenous drugs are very powerful; therefore it is important to check the following *every* time you give drugs:

- drug prescription sheet
- drug
- dose
- route
- time

- rate
- course
- expiry date
- contents (if cloudy or contains sediment, do *not* use).

(7) Draw up and give drugs as instructed. Remember to label syringes carefully.
(8) Some intravenous drugs do not mix well together and crystals can form in the long line. This is why it is very important that saline is given through the line before giving drugs and between each antibiotic.
(9) Give drugs slowly, always maintaining positive pressure.
(10) Saline and water can be kept for 24 hours in the fridge. All other drugs must be discarded after use.
(11) Once drugs have been given, sign the medication sheet. Make notes of any problems or reactions. If any side effects are observed, please contact the hospital immediately.
(12) Dispose of waste material. Glass capsules and sharps, i.e. needles, must be put into a sharps bin.

Try to avoid distraction at all costs:

- Do not answer the phone or door.
- Set aside plenty of time – do not rush.
- Try to get plenty of rest in between drugs as tiredness is a problem. Giving home IVs is demanding.
- Get help with shopping and housework.

Possible complications of giving intravenous drugs

- Allergic reaction
- Blocked line or collapsed vein – inability to give drugs
- Air embolism (air in line – can only cause damage if large amounts of air are injected)
- Thrombosis
- Phlebitis – inflammation/infection
- Infection

Signs of problems

- 'Stiff' arm
- Pain
- Redness

- Swelling
- Inability to inject drugs
- Leakage of drugs

If any of these are observed *do not* give drugs. Contact the hospital.

Table 10.4 *Continued*

Phone numbers
Ward:
Community sister:
Messages: (including times)
Urgent:

Table 10.5 General information on the infusion device.

The infusion device is a device which does not require electricity and is a non-gravity dependent delivery system of antibiotics. The system maintains a constant pressure on the antibiotic within the reservoir (bubble). This continuous pressure coupled with an internal flow metering device produces a known (pre-set) flow rate for the delivery of the contained medication.

Unlike gravity systems, the infusion device frees the patient from equipment such as drip stands and pumps and the setting of flow rates, making the device simple to use. The flow rates are pre-set in a pharmacy providing accurate dosages and pharmacy consistency which gives necessary safety when handling the infusion device.

The infusion device:

● Is small and lightweight and can be hidden under clothing as no other equipment is needed.
● Gives privacy to the patient and helps maintain his/her everyday way-of-life by being free of attachments, enabling the patient to carry on with his/her work, or a child to continue playing.
● Reduces infection risks and the number of complications that arise. The controlled rate prevents drugs being administered too quickly.
● Is sterile, non-pyrogenic and disposable.

---

referrals made by Clare during Jo's admission. Providing Ann (the paediatric community nurse) with this information:

● Facilitates good communication.
● Enables her to be able to quickly contact the relevant individual regarding any particular aspect of Jo's care.
● Ensures that all those involved are kept informed of any change in the management of Jo's treatment whilst at home.

Clare (Jo's primary nurse) has highlighted the fact that a sibling who also had CF died at the age of three years following a severe chest infection (Fig. 10.6). Whilst all CF children and their families receive ongoing support and counselling from specialist social workers, Jo's parents will need additional support throughout the duration of Jo's intravenous antibiotic treatment at home. Including this information on the Community Referral and History Sheet 2 (Fig. 10.6) alerts the paediatric community nursing team to this fact. The Community Referral and History Sheet 1 (Fig. 10.6) informs them that Clare has also contacted Helen Downs (the specialist social worker) to ensure that the family receives the additional support they are likely to require.

Fig. 10.5 The infusion device.

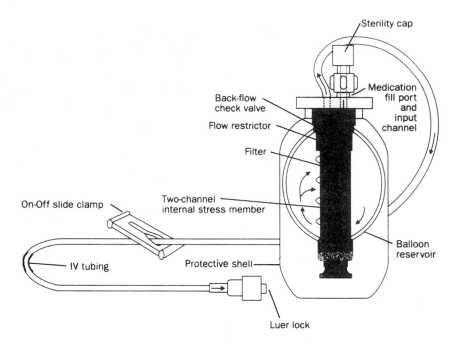

Following Jo's discharge from Beaver ward, Ann (the paediatric community nurse) visited the family home to supervise and support Jo and her mother whilst they administered the lunch-time dose of intravenous antibiotics. At this time Ann completed the remaining section of the Community Referral and History Sheet 2 (Fig. 10.6). This highlights information related to the dynamics of the family and the support available to them. This aspect is particularly important due to the additional time required to administer Jo's intravenous antibiotics, as well as perform her 'usual' level of care. It may be necessary for Jo to be re-admitted or to visit the ward at short notice, and therefore identifying whether the family have their own transport is also a crucial factor that is likely to affect Ann's management of Jo's care if problems arise. Ann has also noted that the family are due to go on holiday at the end of July. As it is important that there is an improvement in Jo's condition prior to that date, regular monitoring to detect an improvement or deterioration will form part of the management of Jo's care.

The Gingerbread Man Assessment Sheet (Fig. 10.7) has been adapted for use in the community. Whilst the section pertaining to Jo's normal Activities of Living contains the same information as that contained within the Assessment Sheet utilized in the hospital setting, the 'On Admission' section has been altered to 'Progress Update'. The information included within the latter incorporates the child and family's perception, as well as the community nurse's assessment, of progress made since the commencement of treatment. Figure 10.7 indicates that Jo's condition has improved since starting intravenous antibiotics. However, it is from the information contained within the 'Progress Update' section of the Gingerbread Man Assessment Sheet (Fig. 10.7) and the Community Referral and History Sheet(s) 1 and 2 that Jo's needs and those of her family can be clearly identified.

In this respect, it can be seen that Ann (the paediatric community nurse) has formulated plans of care that highlight Jo's needs relating to 'Breathing' (Figs 10.8 and 10.9) and 'Safety' (Figs 10.10 and 10.11). These have been devised

Fig. 10.6 (facing page) Case study 5: Community Referral and History Sheet 1 and 2.

Section One: *To be completed by Ward Nurse*	CHILD'S COMMUNITY REFERRAL AND HISTORY SHEET 1	REG NO: 392487
WARD: BEAVER		

Family Name: WILLIAMSON	Date: 2|6|94	Time: 10·00	Nursery/School: GREENWOLD JUNIOR

First Name: JOANNE	Reason for referral: CONTINUATION OF A COURSE OF INTRAVENOUS ANTIBIOTICS AT HOME	
Likes to be called: JO		Names and ages of siblings: THOMAS 5YRS
Age: 8YRS		BEN 11 YRS
DOB: 6-8-86		
Birth weight: 5lb 20Z	Medical Diagnosis: CYSTIC FIBROSIS - CHEST INFECTION	
Religion: C/E Christened: (YES)/NO		

Child's Address: MARYFIELD COTTAGE 30 MARYFIELD LANE RUDDINGTON	What information have parents been given about diagnosis/condition of their child? FULL INFORMATION REGARDING DIAGNOSIS & THE NEED FOR REGULAR TREATMENT. PARENTS HAVE CHOSEN TO CONTINUE CARE AT HOME WHENEVER POSSIBLE	Nursing needs on discharge: SUPERVISION OF THE ADMINISTRATION OF FIRST DOSE OF INTRAVENOUS ANTIBIOTICS GIVEN AT HOME BY ROSEMARY/JO SUPPORT, REASSURANCE & ADVICE RECORDING OF OBSERVATIONS & COLLECTION OF BLOOD SPECIMENS AS PER PROTOCOL
Postcode: NG14 2PJ		

Telephone No: 692471	GP: DR BROOM Address: THE SURGERY RIVERSIDE CLOSE RUDDINGTON	Supplies needed: SYRINGES - 2ml, 5ml + 10ml NEEDLES EXTENSION TUBING BUNGS/CLICK LOCK STREETS SHARPS BOX TEGADERM WATER FOR INJECTION SODIUM CHLORIDE FOR INJECTION HEPFLUSH
Next of Kin: JOHN & ROSEMARY Relationship to child: PARENTS Address if different from above: AS ABOVE		
	Tel No: 684328	
Telephone No: Work: DAD 321489 Home: 692471	Health Visitor: SCHOOL NURSE Address: JUDY GREEN GREENWOLD JUNIOR	
With whom does the child reside: PARENTS, BEN & THOMAS		Referrals made whilst in hospital:

Like to be called: JOHN, ROSEMARY, BEN + TOM	Tel No: 683491	Contact name	Tel No EXT	Title	Date
Relationship to Child: PARENTS + SIBLINGS	Health Centre: THE HEALTH CENTRE Address: BLOOMSBERRY LANE KEYWORTH	SARAH BLUNT	42890	PHYSIO	1|6|94
Who has parental responsibility for this child?: JOHN & ROSEMARY WILLIAMSON		JOHN OLDS	41930	TEACHER	1|6|94
		JUNE BROWN	43270	DIETICIAN	1|6|94
		ANN WINTERS	42670	COMMUNITY NURSE	1|6|94
Telephone number: 692471	Tel No: 528916 Social Worker/other contacts: HELEN DOWNS	HELEN DOWNS	40690	CF SOCIAL WORKER	1|6|94
Child's Ward Nurse/Team: CLARE WELCH	Consultant: DR BROWN	SHEILA DENT	684324	COMMUNITY PHYSIO	2|6|94

Section One (Continued): To be completed by Ward Nurse		Section Two: To be completed by Community Sister	
Appointment given: Date: 12/7/94 Time: 14·00 OPD/~~Ward~~: DR BROWN	Nursing procedures taught to and undertaken by carers/child: * ADMINISTRATION OF INTRAVENOUS ANTIBIOTICS VIA LONGLINE	Why do the parents think the child is being visited: FOR SUPPORT & ADVICE DURING JO'S COURSE OF INTRAVENOUS ANTIBIOTICS	Equipment – Serial Numbers (tick if Disclaimer Form signed) NEBULISER CRXY32481 ✓
Allergies: NONE KNOWN	* ADMINISTRATION OF NEBULISERS & REGULAR PHYSIOTHERAPY * MEASUREMENT OF DAILY PEAK FLOW FOLLOWING PHYSIOTHERAPY		
		What reason does the child give for being visited (if applicable): "TO HELP ME IF I CAN'T GIVE MY MEDICINE INTO THE LINE IN MY ARM"	
Other Information: SIBLING - MATHEW HAD CYSTIC FIBROSIS & DIED AT AGE OF 3YRS IN 1987 FOLLOWING A SEVERE CHEST INFECTION			Other relevant information: * FAMILY HOLIDAY BOOKED FOR THE END OF JULY - COTTAGE IN CORNWALL FOR 2/52. WHOLE FAMILY LOOKING FORWARD TO 'GETTING AWAY'. BEN, JO & TOM VERY EXCITED.
		Social Arrangements: * FAMILY HAS OWN TRANSPORT * JOHN ABLE TO GET TIME OFF WORK AT SHORT NOTICE IF REQUIRED. * PATERNAL GRANDPARENTS LIVE NEARBY & VISIT FREQUENTLY TO ALLOW PARENTS TO GO OUT SOCIALLY. GRANDMOTHER WILL PROVIDE EXTRA ASSISTANCE SUCH AS DOING THE SHOPPING WHILST JO IS UNDERGOING INTRAVENOUS TREATMENT AT HOME. * BEN + TOM ASSIST WITH THE HOUSEHOLD CHORES - TAKE IT IN TURNS TO WASH, DRY & PUT AWAY DISHES & SET TABLE AT MEALTIMES. * BEN HAS LEARNT TO GIVE JO HER PHYSIOTHERAPY & WILL HELP WHEN REQUIRED.	
Current medications & method of administration: CREON CAPSULES MULTIVITAMIN CAPSULES VITAMIN E TABLETS NEBULISED SALBUTAMOL COLOMYCIN NEBULISERS CEPTAZIDINE IV TOBRAMYCIN IV	Procedures not being undertaken by carers/child: * COLLECTION OF BLOOD SPECIMENS AS REQUIRED * OBSERVATIONS OF OXYGEN SATURATION, VITALOGRAPH & WEIGHT ON 7/6/94 & 15/6/94		
		History taken from: (relationship to child) ROSEMARY WILLIAMSON (MOTHER)	

Discharge Date & Time: 3|6|94 11·00	Signature of Nurse referring: C. WELCH	Date: 2|6|94	Signature of Community Nurse taking history A. WINTERS	Date: 3|6|94

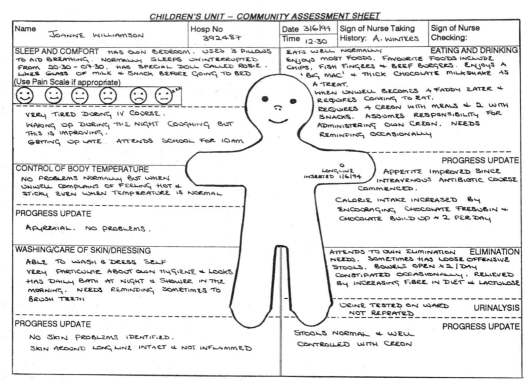

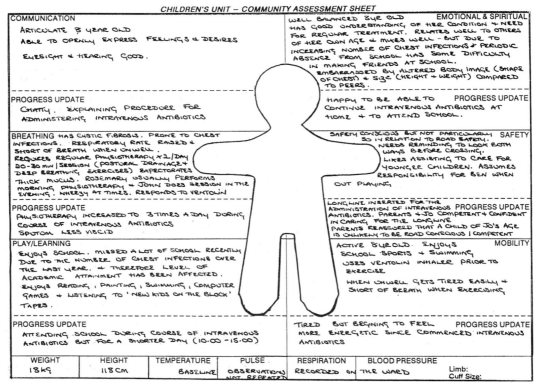

Fig. 10.7 Case study 5: Assessment Sheet (Gingerbread Man).

NURSING CARE PLAN

| NAME | JOANNE WILLIAMSON | | HOSPITAL NO. | 392487 | | AGE | 8 YRS |

ACTIVITY OF LIVING ...... BREATHING

PROBLEM/NEED ...... JO HAS CYSTIC FIBROSIS & IS UNDERGOING TREATMENT FOR A CHEST INFECTION

DATE	TIME	NURSING ACTION	AMEND ACTION TIME, DATE AND SIGN	CHILD/PARENT ACTION	SIGN PARENT AND NURSE
3/6/94	12.45	X RECORD OBSERVATIONS OF OXYGEN SATURATION, VITALOGRAPH (FORCED VITAL CAPACITY + FORCED EXPIRATORY VOLUME¹) + WEIGHT ON 7/6/94 + 15/6/94. LIASE WITH MEDICAL STAFF IF CONDITION NOT IMPROVING		X JO, ROSEMARY + JOHN TO RECORD PEAK FLOW READINGS DAILY FOLLOWING PHYSIOTHERAPY	
		X SEND SPUTUM SAMPLE FOR CULTURE + SENSITIVITY ON 7/6/94 + 15/6/94 FOLLOWING COMPLETION OF THE COURSE OF INTRAVENOUS ANTIBIOTICS		X ROSEMARY TO COLLECT SPUTUM SAMPLE FOLLOWING PHYSIOTHERAPY ON 7/6/94 + 15/6/94	
		X ENCOURAGE PARENTS TO INCREASE PHYSIOTHERAPY TO 3 SESSIONS DURING THE COURSE OF INTRAVENOUS ANTIBIOTICS		X PHYSIOTHERAPY REGIME TO BE INCREASED TO 3 SESSIONS PER DAY. ROSEMARY + JOHN TO SHARE. PARENTS AWARE THAT IN THE EVENT OF ANY DIFFICULTIES THEY SHOULD CONTACT SHEILA DENT (COMMUNITY PHYSIOTHERAPIST) ON TEL: 684324	
		X LIASE WITH COMMUNITY PHYSIOTHERAPIST TO PROVIDE EXTRA SUPPORT DURING JO'S COURSE OF INTRAVENOUS ANTIBIOTICS		X COMMUNITY PHYSIOTHERAPIST WILL VISIT JO AT HOME TO PROVIDE EXTRA SUPPORT + ASSIST WITH PHYSIOTHERAPY	
		X NOTE ANY INCREASE IN COUGH OR BREATHLESSNESS, DECREASE IN PEAKFLOW MEASUREMENTS OR OXYGEN SATURATIONS, REPORT TO MEDICAL STAFF.		X ROSEMARY + JOHN TO REPORT TO COMMUNITY NURSE OR WARD TEAM IF JO'S CONDITION DOES NOT APPEAR TO BE IMPROVING	JO J. WILLIAMSON R. WILLIAMSON
					A. WINTERS

The signature of the parent indicates that this care plan has been negotiated

NURSING CARE PLAN

| NAME | JOANNE WILLIAMSON | | HOSPITAL NO. | 392487 | | AGE | 8 YRS |

ACTIVITY OF LIVING ...... BREATHING

PROBLEM/NEED ...... JO HAS CYSTIC FIBROSIS + IS UNDERGOING TREATMENT FOR A CHEST INFECTION

DATE	TIME	NURSING ACTION	AMEND ACTION TIME, DATE AND SIGN	CHILD/PARENT ACTION	SIGN PARENT AND NURSE
3/6/94	12.45	X REPORT TO MEDICAL STAFF AS APPROPRIATE IF: JO COMPLAINS OF RESTLESSNESS OR BREATHLESSNESS AT NIGHT, OR MORNING HEADACHES, WHICH MAY BE INDICATIVE OF LOW OXYGEN SATURATION AT NIGHT + POOR RESPONSE TO TREATMENT		X JO, ROSEMARY + JOHN TO REPORT TO THE COMMUNITY NURSE IF JO IS INCREASINGLY RESTLESS + UNABLE TO SLEEP, OR IF THERE IS AN INCREASE IN BREATHLESSNESS OR IF SHE EXPERIENCES HEADACHES IN THE MORNING	
		X CHECK NEBULISER SUPPLIES + EQUIPMENT WITH JO + HER PARENTS	3/6/94 13¹⁵ A. WINTERS	X ROSEMARY + JOHN TO ADMINISTER NEBULISERS AS PRESCRIBED.	
				X ROSEMARY + JOHN WILL INFORM THE COMMUNITY NURSE AT THE EARLIEST OPPORTUNITY IF FURTHER SUPPLIES ARE REQUIRED	JO R. WILLIAMSON J. WILLIAMSON
					A. WINTERS.

The signature of the parent indicates that this care plan has been negotiated

Fig. 10.8 Case study 5: Nursing Care Plan – breathing.

NURSING CARE PLAN – PROGRESS UPDATE

NAME	JOANNE WILLIAMSON		HOSPITAL NO. 392487		AGE 8 YRS	
DATE	TIME	ACTIVITY OF LIVING BREATHING	PROBLEM/NEED	JO HAS CYSTIC FIBROSIS & IS UNDER GOING TREATMENT FOR A CHEST INFECTION		SIGN
3/6/94	13·15	NEBULISER SUPPLIES & EQUIPMENT CHECKED				A. WINTERS

Fig. 10.9 Case study 5: Progress Update – breathing.

Fig. 10.10 (below and facing page) Case study 5: Nursing Care Plan – safety.

in conjunction with Jo and her parents. In addition, the negotiated aspects of care and areas of responsibility are clearly identifiable. The importance of ensuring that Jo's parents have access to support and advice is clearly recognized, and the inclusion of contact telephone numbers within care plans assists in this process (Figs 10.12 and 10.13). It should be noted that support is also available from the ward and from other members of the multi-disciplinary team involved in Jo's long-term care. Ensuring that Jo's parents are aware that they can ask for assistance from the paediatric community nurse or for Jo to be readmitted at any time is also of paramount importance and this has also been documented in the plan of care that remains within the home environment (see Fig. 10.8).

NURSING CARE PLAN

NAME	JOANNE WILLIAMSON		HOSPITAL NO. 392487		AGE 8YRS
ACTIVITY OF LIVING	SAFETY		PROBLEM/NEED	JO IS UNDERGOING A COURSE OF INTRAVENOUS ANTIBIOTICS VIA A LONG LINE	

DATE	TIME	NURSING ACTION	AMEND ACTION TIME, DATE AND SIGN	CHILD/PARENT ACTION	SIGN PARENT AND NURSE
3/6/94	12·55	✗ ENSURE LONGLINE IS SECURED SAFELY USING STERISTRIPS & A CLEAR TEGADERM DRESSING SO THAT THE ENTRY SITE MAY BE OBSERVED EASILY FOR SIGNS OF – REDNESS – SWELLING – IRRITATION – LEAKAGE		✗ ROSEMARY WILL REPLACE TEGADERM AS NECESSARY. ADVISED TO TRIM EDGES OF OLD TEGADERM & PLACE REPLACEMENT PIECE OVER THE TOP. ✗ JO & ROSEMARY WILL OBSERVE THE LONGLINE & REPORT ANY PROBLEMS TO THE COMMUNITY NURSE ON CALL OR CONTACT THE WARD IF SHE IS NOT AVAILABLE. ✗ JO & ROSEMARY TO REPORT ANY 'STIFFNESS OF THE LINE' OR BLOCKAGE TO THE COMMUNITY NURSE ON CALL OR CONTACT THE WARD IF SHE IS NOT AVAILABLE	
		✗ OBSERVE LONGLINE & EXTENSION LINE FOR SIGNS OF DAMAGE DUE TO CLAMP		✗ JO & ROSEMARY TO REPORT ANY SIGNS OF DAMAGE TO LONGLINE OR ANY DIFFICULTY WITH THE CLAMP SYSTEM, ADVISED TO CLAMP THE LONGLINE WHEN NOT IN USE & TO RESITE THE CLAMP AFTER EACH USE TO AVOID CONSTANT PRESSURE ON ONE AREA	
		✗ ENSURE THE GREEN BUNG PLACED AT THE END OF THE EXTENSION LINE IS UNDAMAGED & FASTENED SECURELY		✗ JO & ROSEMARY TO CHECK GREEN BUNG IS SECURELY IN PLACE FOLLOWING THE ADMINISTRATION OF INTRAVENOUS ANTIBIOTICS OR HEPFLUSH	
				✗ JO & ROSEMARY TO OBSERVE THE CENTRE OF THE GREEN BUNG FOR SIGNS OF DAMAGE OR 'BULGING' & REPLACE IF NECESSARY USING STERILE GLOVES	JO R. WILLIAMSON J. WILLIAMSON A. WINTERS
				The signature of the parent indicates that this care plan has been negotiated	

NURSING CARE PLAN

NAME	JOANNE WILLIAMSON		HOSPITAL NO. 392487		AGE 8YRS
ACTIVITY OF LIVING SAFETY			PROBLEM/NEED JO IS UNDERGOING A COURSE OF INTRAVENOUS ANTIBIOTICS VIA A LONGLINE		

DATE	TIME	NURSING ACTION	AMEND ACTION TIME, DATE AND SIGN	CHILD/PARENT ACTION	SIGN PARENT AND NURSE
3/6/94	12.55	X OBSERVE THE ADMINISTRATION OF THE FIRST DOSE OF INTRAVENOUS ANTIBIOTICS GIVEN AT HOME BY JO & ROSEMARY	3/6/94 13.30 A.WINTERS	X JO & ROSEMARY TO ADMINISTER INTRAVENOUS ANTIBIOTICS & HEPFLUSH AS PER DRUG CHART & PROTOCOLS	
				X JO & ROSEMARY TO SIGN DRUG CHART FOLLOWING THE ADMINISTRATION OF EACH DOSE OF ANTIBIOTICS	
		X ENSURE JO & HER PARENTS ARE AWARE OF THE CORRECT DISPOSAL OF SHARPS & WASTE PRODUCTS		X JO, ROSEMARY & JOHN FULLY AWARE OF & WILL ADHERE TO POLICIES REGARDING THE SAFE DISPOSAL OF SHARPS & WASTE PRODUCTS	
		X IN VIEW OF LONGLINE INSITU LIASE WITH SCHOOL NURSE IN CASE OF DIFFICULTIES OR PROBLEMS OCCURING AT SCHOOL			
		X CHECK SUPPLIES FOR THE ADMINISTRATION OF INTRAVENOUS ANTIBIOTICS	3/6/94 13.15 A.WINTERS	X ROSEMARY TO INFORM COMMUNITY NURSE AT THE EARLIEST OPPORTUNITY IF FURTHER SUPPLIES ARE REQUIRED & TO REPORT ANY PROBLEMS OR DIFFICULTIES WITH THE INFUSION DEVICE TO THE MANUFACTURERS & THE COMMUNITY NURSE	
		X LIASE WITH MEDICAL STAFF RE: ANY SIDE EFFECTS FROM ANTIBIOTICS		X ROSEMARY & JOHN AWARE OF POTENTIAL SIDE EFFECTS SUCH AS A RED RASH, NAUSEA OR DIARRHOEA (SEE PARENT INFORMATION SHEET: ANTIBIOTICS USED IN CYSTIC FIBROSIS) & WILL REPORT TO THE COMMUNITY NURSE OR WARD TEAM IF THEY OCCUR OR IF THEY ARE CONCERNED	Jo R.Williamson J.Williamson A.WINTERS
				The signature of the parent indicates that this care plan has been negotiated	

NURSING CARE PLAN

NAME	JOANNE WILLIAMSON		HOSPITAL NO. 392487		AGE 8YRS
ACTIVITY OF LIVING SAFETY			PROBLEM/NEED JO IS UNDERGOING A COURSE OF INTRAVENOUS ANTIBIOTICS VIA A LONGLINE		

DATE	TIME	NURSING ACTION	AMEND ACTION TIME, DATE AND SIGN	CHILD/PARENT ACTION	SIGN PARENT AND NURSE
3/6/94	12.55	X COLLECT BLOOD SPECIMENS TO CHECK TOBRAMYCIN LEVELS AS INSTRUCTED BY MEDICAL STAFF. DUE TO BE TAKEN ON 7/6/94. LIASE WITH MEDICAL STAFF RE: ANY ALTERATION IN DRUG DOSAGE		X JO & HER PARENTS AWARE THAT FINGER PRICK SAMPLES OF BLOOD WILL NEED TO BE TAKEN DURING THE COURSE OF HER INTRAVENOUS ANTIBIOTICS	
		X REMOVE LONGLINE ON 15/6/94 FOLLOWING COMPLETION OF THE COURSE OF INTRAVENOUS ANTIBIOTICS. REFER TO MEDICAL STAFF IF ANY DIFFICULTIES EXPERIENCED.			Jo R.Williamson J.Williamson A.WINTERS
				The signature of the parent indicates that this care plan has been negotiated	

<u>NURSING CARE PLAN – PROGRESS UPDATE</u>

NAME JOANNE WILLIAMSON		HOSPITAL NO 392487	AGE 8 YRS
DATE	TIME	ACTIVITY OF LIVING SAFETY .... PROBLEM/NEED JO IS UNDERGOING A COURSE OF INTRAVENOUS ANTIBIOTICS VIA A LONGLINE	SIGN
3/6/94	13.15	SUPPLIES & EQUIPMENT FOR THE ADMINISTRATION OF ANTIBIOTICS CHECKED	A. WINTERS
	13.30	INTRAVENOUS ANTIBIOTICS ADMINISTERED COMPETENTLY BY JO & ROSEMARY. LONGLINE	JO
		PATENT. NO SIGNS OF INFLAMMATION OR LEAKAGE.	R. Williamson
			A. WINTERS

Fig. 10.11 Case study 5: Progress Update – safety.

<u>NURSING CARE PLAN</u>

NAME JOANNE WILLIAMSON		HOSPITAL NO. 392487		AGE 8 YRS
ACTIVITY OF LIVING EMOTIONAL / SPIRITUAL		PROBLEM/NEED JO IS UNDERGOING A COURSE OF INTRAVENOUS ANTIBIOTICS AT HOME & JO & HER PARENTS REQUIRE SUPPORT		
DATE	TIME	NURSING ACTION	AMEND ACTION TIME, DATE AND SIGN	CHILD/PARENT ACTION	SIGN PARENT AND NURSE
3/6/94	13.10	X ENSURE JO & HER PARENTS ARE AWARE OF HOW TO CONTACT THE COMMUNITY NURSE	3/6/94 13.10 X A. WINTERS .	X ROSEMARY & JOHN POSSESS CONTACT NUMBERS & UNDERSTAND THE BLEEP SYSTEM	
		X PROVIDE SUPPORT BY ADMINISTERING JO'S INTRAVENOUS ANTIBIOTICS AS PRE-ARRANGED WITH JOHN & ROSEMARY		X ROSEMARY & JOHN AWARE THAT THE COMMUNITY NURSE WILL ADMINISTER INTRAVENOUS ANTIBIOTICS IF ARRANGED IN ADVANCE & THAT JO CAN BE RE-ADMITTED IF THEY EXPERIENCE DIFFICULTIES OR IF AN UNEXPECTED EVENT OR FAMILY CRISIS OCCURS	JO J. WILLIAMSON R. WILLIAMSON A. WINTERS

The signature of the parent indicates that this care plan has been negotiated

Fig. 10.12 Case study 5: Nursing Care Plan – emotional/spiritual.

<u>NURSING CARE PLAN – PROGRESS UPDATE</u>

NAME JOANNE WILLIAMSON		HOSPITAL NO 392487	AGE 8 YRS
DATE	TIME	ACTIVITY OF LIVING EMOTIONAL/SPIRITUAL PROBLEM/NEED JO & HER PARENTS NEED SUPPORT	SIGN
3/6/94	13.10	CONTACT TELEPHONE NUMBERS GIVEN TO ROSEMARY & JOHN. BLEEP SYSTEM EXPLAINED	
			A. WINTERS

Fig. 10.13 Case study 5: Progress Update – emotional/spiritual.

The care of a child with a chronic illness such as cystic fibrosis continues beyond periodic hospital admissions or the facilitation of courses of treatment within the home environment. It involves frequent attendance at follow-up clinics for review by the multi-disciplinary team and ongoing support and counselling from specialist social workers. However, the role of a specialist nurse or link nurse is of paramount importance in maintaining a co-ordinated approach to care, and in facilitating good communication between hospital-based and community-based professionals (Table 10.6).

Table 10.6 The role of the cystic fibrosis link facilitator.

(1) To act as a resource person in an advisory/liaison capacity on all aspects of CF care.

(2) To be responsible for organizing and maintaining the education and training programme for families wishing to undertake home IV therapy.

(3) To effectively liaise on a regular basis with the community paediatric nursing team regarding the nursing care of CF patients in hospital and at home.

(4) To attend, at regular intervals, the Cystic Fibrosis Out-patient Clinic (in particular post-clinic meetings) to be updated on patients attending clinic.

(5) To be in attendance at shared-clinics to offer support and advice to families and other health professionals.

(6) To liaise with the manufacturers of the infusion device to help develop and promote the home IV service.

Offering families the opportunity to care for their child at home and providing the vital support to enable them to do so is particularly important for children with chronic or life-threatening illnesses. Undoubtedly this assists in maintaining as much normality as possible for the child and family, and enchances the quality of life that they experience [43].

References

1. Griffiths, R. (1988) *Community Care: Agenda For Action*. HMSO, London.
2. Department of Health (1989) *Caring For People*. HMSO, London.
3. Capes, M. (1955) The Child in Hospital. *Bulletin of the World Health Organization*, **12**, 427–70.
4. Ministry of Health (1959) *The Welfare of Children in Hospital* (Platt Report). HMSO, London.
5. Report of the Committee on Child Health Services (1976) *Fit For The Future* (Court Report). HMSO, London.
6. Audit Commission (1986) *Making a Reality of Community Care: A Report*. HMSO, London.
7. Department of Health (1991) *Welfare of Children and Young People in Hospital*. HMSO, London.
8. Belson, P. (1981) Alternatives to hospital care. *Nursing*, **23**, 1015–16.
9. While, A.E. (1991) An Evaluation of a Paediatric Home Care Scheme. *Journal of Advanced Nursing*, **16**, 1413–21.

10. Downie, R. (1991) *Patterns of Hospital Medical Staffing: Paediatrics.* HMSO, London.
11. Lefebvre, F., Veilleux, A. & Bard, H. (1982) Early discharge of low birth weight infants. *Archives of Disease in Childhood*, **57**, 511–13.
12. Brooken, D., Kumar, S., Brown, L.P., Butts, P., Finkler, S.A. & Glakewell-Sachs, S. (1986) A randomised clinical trial of early discharge and follow up of very low birth weight infants. *New England Journal of Medicine*, **315** (15), 934–9.
13. Dryden, S. (1989) Care in the Community. *Paediatric Nursing*, **1** (7), 19–20.
14. Dryden, S. (1989) Paediatric Medicine in the Community. *Paediatric Nursing*, **1** (8), 17–18.
15. Catchpole, A. (1985) *Community Paediatric Nursing Services in England.* Unpublished research, Department of Management and Business Studies, Oxford Polytechnic, Oxford.
16. Atwell, J.D. & Gow, M.A. (1985) Paediatric trained district nurse in the community: expensive luxury or economic necessity? *British Medical Journal* **291**, 227–9.;
17. Audit Commission (1993) *Children First: A Study of Hospital Services.* HMSO, London.
18. Chamberlain, T.M., Lehman, M.E., Groh, M.J., Munroe, W.P. & Reinders, T.P. (1988) Cost Analysis of a Home Intravenous Antibiotic Programme. *American Journal of Hospital Pharmacy*, **45** (2), 2341–5.
19. Donati, M.A., Guenette, G. & Auerbach, H. (1987) Prospective Controlled Study of Home and Hospital Therapy of Cystic Fibrosis Pulmonary Disease. *Journal of Pediatrics*, **11** (1), 28–30.
20. Rutter, M. (1982) *Maternal Deprivation Re-assessed.* Penguin, Harmondsworth.
21. Bowlby, J. (1952) *Maternal Care and Mental Health*, 2nd ed. World Health Organization, Geneva.
22. Bowlby, J. (1953) *Child Care and the Growth of Love.* Pelican, Harmondsworth.
23. Robertson, J. (1970) *Young Chiildren in Hospital.* Tavistock, London.
24. Butler, N.R. & Golding, J. (1986) *From Birth to Five.* Pergamon, Oxford.
25. Douglas, J. (1993) *Psychology and Nursing Children.* Macmillan, London.
26. Muller, D.J., Harris, P.J., Wattley, L. & Taylor, J.D. (1992) *Nursing Children: Psychology, research and practice*, 2nd ed. Chapman & Hall, London.
27. Couriel, J.M. & Davies, P. (1988) Costs and benefits of a community special care baby service. *British Medical Journal*, **296**, 1043–6.
28. Campbell, J.R., Scaife, J.M. & Johnstone, J.M.S. (1988) Psychological effects of day case surgery compared with in patient surgery. *Archives of Disease in Childhood*, **63**, 415–17.
29. Sainsbury, C.P.Q., Gray, O.P., Cleary, J., Davies, M.M. & Rowlandson, P.H. (1986) Care by parents of their children in hospital. *Archives of Disease in Childhood*, **61**, 612–15.
30. Cleary, J., Gray, O.P., Hall, D., Rowlandson, P.H., Sainsbury, C.P.Q. & Davies, M.M. (1986) Parental involvement in the lives of children in hospital. *Archives of Disease in Childhood*, **61**, 779–87.
31. Edwardson, S.R. (1983) The choice between hospital and home care for terminally ill children. *Nursing Research*, **32**, 29–34.
32. Campbell, M. (1987) Children with on-going health needs. *Nursing, Third Series*, **23**, 871–5.

33. Martin, F.R. (1975) The nurse's role in the home care unit. *Nursing Mirror*, **141**, 70–72.
34. Carlson, P., Simacek, M., Henry, W. & Martinson, I. (1985) A model home care program for the dying child. *Issues in Comprehensive Pediatric Nursing*, **8** (1–6), 113–27.
35. Martinson, I., Moldow, G., Armstrong, G., Henry, W., Nesbitt, M. & Kersey, J. (1987) Home care for the child dying of cancer. *Research Nursing Health*, **77** (1), 11–16.
36. Walsh, A. (1987) Death always a threat . . . sometimes a reality. In: *Childhood Cancer – A Nursing Overview* (eds S. Maul Mellot & J. Adams). Jones & Bartlett, Boston.
37. Dufour, D.F. (1989) Home or hospital care for the child with end stage cancer: effects on the family. *Issues in Comprehensive Pediatric Nursing*, **12** (5), 371–83.
38. Martinson, I., Armstrong, G., Geis, D., Anglim, M., Granseth, E., MacInnis, H., Kersey, J. & Nesbitt, M. (1978) Home care for children dying of cancer. *Paediatrics*, **62**, 106–13.
39. Fradd, E. (1990) Setting up a Paediatric Community Nursing Service. *Senior Nurse*, **10** (7), 4–7.
40. Dryden, S. (1986) Home Healing. *Community Outlook*, October, 25–6.
41. Royal College of Nursing (1993) *Buying Paediatric Community Nursing*. RCN, London.
42. Stower, S. (1991) A Quality Service for Children in the Out-patient Setting. *International Journal of Health Care Quality Assurance*, **4** (6), 4–9.
43. Armour, S. (1991) Andrew. In: *This Is Our Child* (eds A. Cooper & V. Harpin). Oxford University Press, Oxford.

Appendix 1
Parent Information Leaflets

Introduction

There are in excess of 250 specifically designed information sheets available for parents and families within the Children's Unit in Nottingham. They provide information in relation to a wide variety of issues including:

- a child's illness and treatment;
- forthcoming procedures or investigations; and
- continuing care at home following discharge from hospital.

All the Parent Information Sheets are written in easily understandable terms and diagrams or pictures are incorporated as appropriate to aid understanding.

The examples included within this appendix relate to:

- Pyloric stenosis
- Hydrocele operation
- Control of a high temperature*
- If your child has a febrile convulsion*
- Apnoea alarm*
- Hypospadias repair – care of your son*
- Hypospadias repair (with catheter) – care of your son*
- Antibiotics used in cystic fibrosis*

The Parent Information Sheets may be:

- Given to parents in the Children's Out-patient Department following the identification of a need for their child to have an operation, sent to them prior to the planned admission of their child or given to them during the initial admission period. See for example 'Hydrocele operation'.
- Given to parents following initial diagnosis or prior to various procedures. See for example 'Pyloric stenosis'.
- Given to parents during their child's hospital admission as a means of providing information regarding the care of their child following discharge. See for example 'Hypospadias repair – care of your son'.
- Given to parents during the child's admission as a source of information or prior to discharge from the Children's Accident and Emergency

* These Information Sheets relate to/have been referred to in one of the case studies.

Department. See for example 'Control of a high temperature' and 'If your child has a febrile convulsion'.

It is intended that all Parent Information Sheets will be freely available within Family Resource areas situated within the Children's Out-patient Departments. Whilst Parent Information Sheets *do not* and *should not* be used to replace verbal explanations or discussion, they act as a useful source of reference for parents and families, and reinforce verbal information given by professionals. They also act as a means of assisting with discharge planning. See for example 'Apnoea alarm', utilized within case study 2.

It should be noted that whilst the majority of the Parent Information Sheets are written in general terms, several have the facility to be individualized. See for example 'Hypospadias repair (with catheter) – care of your son'. All the Parent Information Sheets are reviewed and updated on a regular basis, with additional ones being constantly added to those already available.

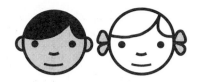

PARENT INFORMATION SHEET

PYLORIC STENOSIS

WARD: . . . .

When you come into hospital with your baby and you are told that your baby has pyloric stenosis, you may find this leaflet useful to help you understand what the doctor has told you.

If you have any questions, please do not hesitate to talk to the nurse looking after your baby.

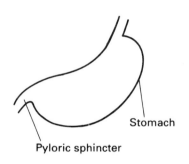

What is pyloric stenosis?

Pyloric stenosis is a thickening and narrowing of the muscle called the pyloric sphincter which is at the lower end of the stomach (see diagram). This causes what is known as projectile or forceful vomiting following feeds. Your baby may appear to be miserable, hungry and he/she may lose weight.

How will the doctors know what is wrong?

The nurse looking after your baby will observe him/her feeding and the doctor will do what is called a 'test feed' – whilst your baby is feeding the doctor will feel and look at your baby's tummy. The doctor will be able to feel the thickened muscle.

Sometimes the doctor will do an ultrasound – a scan using high frequency sound waves that produces a picture of your baby's tummy on a screen (the same kind of scan that pregnant mothers have).

How is it corrected?

Your baby will need a minor operation to correct the narrow, thickened muscle. The doctor will explain the procedure to you. However, if you have any further questions or worries, please ask the nurse looking after your baby.

You may be able to accompany your baby to the anaesthetic room and go with the nurse to collect him/her from the recovery room after the operation. If you wish to do so, please speak to the nurse looking after your baby.

Before the operation

The doctor will take a small sample of blood from your baby to check that the content of his/her blood is normal.

Your baby will not be able to feed prior to the operation, so an intravenous infusion or 'drip' will be started. A tube (called a naso-gastric tube) will be passed through his/her nose into the stomach so as to remove any stale milk.

After the operation

When your baby returns from theatre, he/she will have either an elasto-plast or a small dressing on his/her tummy.

Your baby may still have the 'drip' and naso-gastric tube in place. These will be removed once your baby is feeding normally.

Feeding

The re-introduction of feeds varies according to your baby's doctor. The doctor and nurse looking after your baby will be able to give you more details. However, most babies commence feeding gradually.

It is not uncommon for some babies to vomit a little after the operation.

Discharge home

When your baby is feeding normally, you will be able to go home. This is usually about 48–72 hours after the operation.

Before you go home you will be given an appointment for your baby to have a check-up in the Children's Out-patient Department. This is usually about six weeks after your baby's operation.

If you have any problems or queries when you return home, please do not hesitate to telephone the ward on:

TEL:

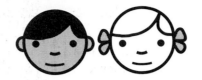

PARENT INFORMATION SHEET

HYDROCELE OPERATION

WARD: ....

Your son has had an operation to repair a hydrocele.

Pain or discomfort

Calpol or paracetamol-based medicine can be given. Cotton underpants will give support if the scrotum is swollen.

Dressing and baths

The plaster over the operation site should be kept clean and dry for one week. During this time showers or shallow baths may be given. If the plaster becomes wet, remove it, dry the wound and re-apply a clean plaster. The plaster may be removed after one week. There are no stitches to come out as these will have dissolved away.

Diet and drinks

Your son can eat and drink normally the day after the operation. If he is going home on the day of operation he may have something light to eat, such as toast or cereals, as he may feel sick if he has too much too soon.

Play and activity

Your child will benefit from extra rest for the next two to three days and then will gradually start doing more. However, he *should not* ride a bike, straddle toys, play games such as football or take part in PE or games at school or go swimming for the next three to four weeks. He can go back to school when he is feeling no discomfort – usually after seven to ten days. Please let the school/playgroup know your child has had an operation.

An appointment will be made for your son to see the doctor in clinic in approximately six weeks. If before your clinic appointment is due you are at all worried or concerned about your son's operation or condition, please do not hesitate to seek help. Either telephone the ward on ....
ext. .... and ask to speak to ....,
your primary nurse, or speak to the nurse in charge, or contact your GP.

PARENT INFORMATION SHEET

CONTROL OF A HIGH TEMPERATURE

WARD: . . . .

A high temperature usually indicates infection. Any child with a temperature higher than 38.5°C should be seen by your family doctor if it persists for more than 24 hours.

In younger children (less than one year) infection may progress rapidly, and you should seek medical help early, either through your family doctor or the casualty department.

Risk of convulsion with temperature

Children between six months and five years are at risk of developing a convulsion with a high temperature. Prevention is better than cure, and measures should include the following:

(1) Take off most of your child's clothes so he/she can lose heat through the skin. *Do not* wrap your child in blankets or duvets. If your child is up and about, a vest and a nappy is appropriate. If in bed, a light sheet only is acceptable.
(2) Give your child regular medication (as directed on the bottle) to help bring the temperature down. Paracetamol or Ibuprofen are appropriate and are available over the counter. Asprin is *not* appropriate.
(3) Give your child plenty to drink, for example squash or water. Do not worry about food if your child does not feel like eating.

If you are at all worried about your child's condition, call your family doctor.

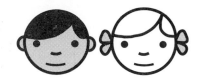

PARENT INFORMATION SHEET

IF YOUR CHILD HAS A CONVULSION

WARD: ....

A convulsion is a fit and is also sometimes called a seizure. If your child has a fit:

(1) Lie your child on the left side with his/her face turned downwards so that if there is anything in the mouth your child will not choke.
(2) Lie your child on a surface where he/she cannot be hurt – on the carpet, floor or bed.
(3) Do not leave your child.
(4) Do not try to force anything into your child's mouth.
(5) Do not slap or shake your child.
(6) If your child has a temperature this may have caused the fit. Try and bring the temperature down by removing clothing.

The fit usually stops by itself in a few minutes – you should let your GP know afterwards.

Your doctor may have prescribed a drug which can be given into the bottom (Stesolid) if the fit has lasted longer than five minutes. If the fit has not stopped within ten minutes, call an ambulance and bring your child to the nearest hospital Accident and Emergency Department.

You can always telephone the ward for advice.

If you have not been given medicine and the fit does not stop after a few minutes then call an ambulance to bring your child to the nearest Accident and Emergency Department.

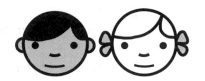

PARENT INFORMATION SHEET

APNOEA ALARM

(sometimes known as respiration monitor or breathing monitor)

WARD: . . . .

This leaflet *must* be read carefully before you go home.
Please ask if you have any queries or if you are unsure about using the apnoea alarm.

What is an apnoea alarm?

The apnoea alarm monitors each breath that your baby takes.
If your baby stops breathing and has an apnoea attack, the alarm will sound to alert you. It is important to realize that the alarm *does not prevent* an apnoea attack but *alerts* you if this occurs.
The apnoea alarm should be used whenever your baby sleeps – not just at night.

How does it work?

The sensor sends a signal to the apnoea alarm every time your baby takes a breath.
As your baby takes a breath, a light on the monitor will flash and you will hear a click.
The alarm should be set at 20 seconds – this means that if your baby does not take a breath for a period of 20 seconds the alarm will sound.

How to attach the sensor to your baby

(1)   Ensure that your baby's abdomen is clean and dry.
(2)   Place the sensor where your baby's abdomen moves the most when he/she takes a breath (see diagram). However, not all babies are the same, so you may need to experiment to find the best place to attach the sensor in order to prevent false alarms. To prevent the lead from the sensor becoming entangled around your baby's neck or fingers, *it is very important* when applying the sensor that the lead is taped twice using hypo-allergenic tape (see diagram on facing page above) and then threaded through your baby's clothing.

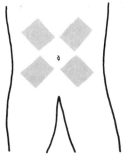

The shaded areas are suggested sites for placing the sensor.

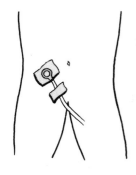

(3) The sensor can be removed when your baby is awake and re-applied before he/she goes to sleep.

Setting the alarm

(1) Plug the sensor into the inlet socket of the monitor (see diagram below). Twist it slightly to make sure it is secure, but do not push too hard.

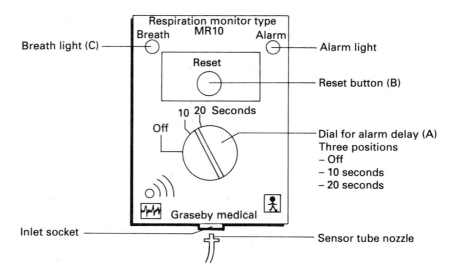

(2) Turn the alarm dial (A) to 20 seconds.
(3) Press and hold down the reset button (B).
(4) When your baby takes a breath, a click will be heard and the breath light (C) will flash.

If the battery is low

The breath light (C) will flash red instead of green if the battery is low. At this point the battery must be replaced as soon as possible.
If this is ignored, a non-resetable audible alarm will sound to indicate an exhausted battery.
The alarm uses one 9V battery.

If the monitor alarms

Go to your baby as quickly as possible, *but do not panic*.

If the monitor is still alarming

● Press the reset button.
● Look at your baby. Check the baby's colour. Open his/her clothes – is he/she breathing?

If your baby is not breathing   Carry out resuscitation as demonstrated by the doctor and on the video *The Breath of Life* which you watched before you left the hospital.

Emergency action   Look at your baby's chest – is he/she breathing? Pick the baby up and gently shake him/her to establish whether or not he/she is unconscious.

If unresponsive, the airway may be obstructed. Use a finger to remove foreign matter that is visible in the mouth. Use a combination of back blows and gravity to dislodge solid foreign matter from lower airways and move it into the mouth.

(1) 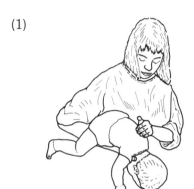 Turn the baby onto his/her front and firmly tap his/her back two to three times to dislodge any mucus blocking the throat.

(2) 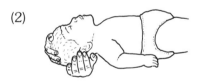 Place the baby on his/her back on a table or any other firm surface. If the baby does not gasp and breathe:

- Support the back of the neck, tilt the head backwards and hold the chin upwards. Open your mouth wide and breathe in.

(3) 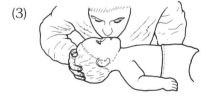 • Seal your lips around the baby's mouth and nose. Breathe gently into his/her lungs until the chest rises.

(4) 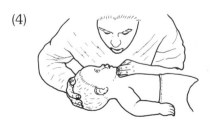 • Remove your mouth to allow the air to come out and let the baby's chest fall.
- Repeat gentle inflations a little faster than your normal breathing rate, removing your mouth after each breath – approximately 30 times per minute.

The baby should begin to breathe within a minute or so.

(5) 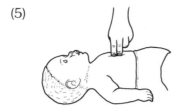 If your baby does not begin to breathe begin cardiac message. With two fingers, gently press your baby's chest in the centre just below the nipples, at a rate of 90/100 times per minute.

If the audible alarm has stopped but the alarm light is flashing
Your baby did not take a breath for the set alarm limit (20 seconds) or the monitor failed to sense one, *but* the baby has taken a breath since.
Press the reset button to cancel the alarm light and observe your baby's breathing for a short period.

If the monitor alarms frequently
This may be due to:

- Incorrect positioning of the sensor.
- Dislodgement of the sensor.
- Monitor failure.

Remember that as your baby becomes more mobile the alarm function will be hindered.

Monitor failure and faults

- Check the battery is fitted correctly. If you are in doubt about the state of the battery, change it. Always keep a supply of spare batteries in the house.
- If no breath signal is registering then:

  (1) Check the sensor is firmly inserted into the socket.
  (2) Replace the tape and reposition the sensor.
  (3) Change the sensor.

You will have been provided with a supply of sensors and tape when you collect the alarm. If you require more supplies, or if the monitor fails to function, or if you have any queries, contact:

Children's Intensive Care Unit
E Floor
East Block
Queen's Medical Centre
Nottingham
Tel: (0115) 9249924 ext 43422

Linby Ward
H Block
Nottingham City Hospital
Nottingham
Tel: (0115) 9691169 ext 46459

Please note

Whilst the monitor is in your possession you are held responsible for it. Prior to discharge you will be asked to sign a form accepting this responsibility.

When you are no longer using the monitor, please return it to us as soon as possible as the demand for such pieces of equipment is great.

Often the doctor may stipulate a time period, usually until your baby is six months of age.

Checklist

Sign and date

(1) Parents seen by doctor and resuscitation
      technique demonstrated.
(2) Video *The Breath of Life* seen.
(3) Indemnity form signed and date for return
      established.
(4) Five sensors and one roll of tape issued.
(5) Functioning and setting up of alarm
      demonstrated and explained.

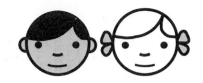

PARENT INFORMATION SHEET

HYPOSPADIAS REPAIR (WITH CATHETER)
CARE OF YOUR SON

WARD: . . . .

. . . . has a catheter following his operation. The catheter will need to stay in place for . . . . days.

For the catheter to drain and work properly . . . . needs to drink more than he normally does.

The dressing around the penis should stay dry if the catheter is working properly. If it becomes wet, please contact the ward nurses for advice. Do not touch the sticky tape as this is all that holds the catheter in place. If it begins to fall off, stick more plaster on top. If you are worried, please contact the ward nurses for advice.

Urine should be draining all the time along the catheter and it should be clear. If it becomes cloudy encourage . . . . to drink more to help clear it. If the urine becomes blood-stained please contact the ward nurses for advice. The catheter bag needs to be changed every third day as you were shown in hospital. Loose fitting clothing is best to prevent a kink in the catheter.

You were given laxatives for your son so that he can open his bowels every day without straining. The medicine may make his stools loose; do not worry unless it happens more than once a day. Again, telephone the ward nurses for advice if you are concerned. Antibiotics, if prescribed, should be given as instructed.

. . . . needs to have his catheter removed on . . . . Please return to the ward between 9 and 11 AM on that day. Once the catheter has been removed and . . . . has passed urine, you can go home. We will arrange a clinic appointment for six weeks after your son's operation.

If you have any queries, please do not hesitate to phone the ward and speak to your primary nurse . . . . or the nurse in charge.

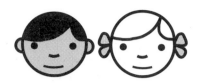

PARENT INFORMATION SHEET

HYPOSPADIAS REPAIR – CARE OF YOUR SON

WARD: . . . .

Eating and drinking

Try and encourage your son to drink. Offer him more drinks than normal for the first three days that he is home. This will encourage him to pass urine.

Wound care

The penis may look red and swollen for up to three weeks following the operation. During this time bathing once or twice a day for a week will be helpful as long as the wound is gently dried. Do not add bubble bath, etc. to the water.
The stitches are dissolvable so they do not need to be removed.

Discomfort

It may be necessary for some pain relief to be given during the first few days. Calpol or another paracetamol-based medicine are suitable.

Clothing

Pants and trousers may be worn when comfortable. Loose fitting clothing is preferable, e.g. boxer shorts, tracksuit bottoms.

Play

Until three to four weeks after the operation your son *must not* ride a bike, play football, climb, take part in PE or sit on toys that he straddles.

School

Your son should be able to go back to school/nursery when he no longer has any discomfort. This is usually after about two weeks.

Clinic

An appointment will be made for approximately six weeks after the operation. If you have any queries, please do not hesitate to phone the ward and speak to your Primary Nurse .... or the nurse in charge.

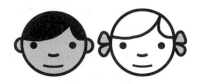

PARENT INFORMATION SHEET

ANTIBIOTICS USED IN CYSTIC FIBROSIS

Introduction

In theory, antibiotics should work by 'selective toxicity'. This means that they should destroy the infecting organism without harming the patient. In practice, the use of highly potent anti-bacterial agents is limited by the adverse side-effects that they could inflict upon the patient. Consequently, we have to balance the potency of an antibiotic against the adverse effects that it may induce. This general concept is equally applicable to patients suffering from cystic fibrosis.

Mode of action

Essentially, all antibiotics work in one of three ways:

(1) They burst the cell wall of the bacteria, e.g. penicillins.
(2) They prevent replication of the bacteria, e.g. erythromycin.
(3) They disrupt metabolism within the bacteria, e.g. sulphonamides.

In any event, each mode of action would eventually result in the death of the bacteria and hopefully eradication of the infection.

Bacteria associated with infection in cystic fibrosis

Three main groups of bacteria are known to be commonly associated with chest infections in patients who have cystic fibrosis. The appropriate antibiotics that are active against the suspected bacteria are consequently used to counter infection.

Haemophilus species
Amoxycillin (Amoxil) – a penicillin that may cause nausea, diarrhoea, indigestion and skin rashes.
Co-trimoxazole (Septrin) – a sulphonamide that may cause nausea, vomiting, diarrhoea, skin rashes and a sore tongue.

Staphylococcus aureus
Flucloxacillin (Floxapen) – a penicillin that may cause nausea, vomiting and skin rashes. Very rarely, jaundice may develop.
Erythromycin – a macrolide that is often used for people who are allergic to

penicillins. Side-effects include nausea, vomiting, diarrhoea and abdominal pain.

Pseudamonas species

Tobramycin (Nebcin) and gentamicin (Genticin) – aminoglycoside antibiotics which can produce adverse effects upon the kidneys and the ear. Dizziness, vertigo, tinnitus and deafness can result as well as kidney dysfunction. Nausea, vomiting, diarrhoea, fever and skin rashes may also result.

Azlocillin (Securopen) – a penicillin that may produce nausea, vomiting, diarrhoea and skin rashes. It can also cause pain at the site of injection as well as disturbing the normal blood picture.

Ceftazidime (Fortum) – a cephalosporin that can cause nausea, vomiting, diarrhoea, fever and skin rashes. It can cause pain at the site of injection but may also cause taste changes, thrush and pins and needles.

Ciprofloxacin (Ciproxin) – a quinoline antibiotic that can cause nausea, vomiting, diarrhoea, dyspepsia and abdominal upset. It can also cause restlessness, dizziness, headaches, shaking, aching joints and blurred vision.

It should be remembered that all of the previously mentioned adverse effects are usually minor or fairly rare. However, since a drug is a substance that is foreign to the body, it may produce an 'idiosyncratic reaction', i.e. it may produce an unexpected, untoward effect that could not have been predicted. Fortunately, these idiosyncratic reactions are extremely rare.

Conclusion

In general, antibiotics will be given that are appropriate to the known or suspected infecting organism. Side-effects may occur, but at normal doses these should be minor and hopefully rare. However, if you suspect that you/your child is experiencing a side-effect from a particular antibiotic, you should seek further advice from a doctor, nurse or pharmacist.

Appendix 2
Ward Information Leaflets

Introduction

Information Sheets provide parents and families with information concerning the ward/department to which their child is to be admitted. They may be:

- Handed to parents in the Children's Out-patient Department or sent to them prior to the planned admission of their child.
- Handed to parents in the Children's Accident and Emergency Department in the event of an emergency admission.
- Handed to parents if their child is to be transferred to another area, i.e. from the Children's Intensive Care Unit to a ward area.

Each individual ward/department has their own Information Sheets, highlighting those aspects that they consider to be important for their particular area. As with all Parent Information Sheets, these are updated on a regular basis.

The examples included within this appendix relate to:

- A medical ward (E37).
- A surgical ward (E40).
- The Children's Intensive Care Unit.

It can be seen that those related to the medical and surgical wards are more detailed than that pertaining to the Children's Intensive Care Unit. The purpose of the latter is to allay some of the fear and anxiety attached to intensive care areas, without providing excessive information to parents and families at what is usually a highly stressful time. It should also be noted that in respect of those related to the surgical ward, different versions have been devised for planned and emergency admissions.

PARENT INFORMATION SHEET

WELCOME TO E37

Welcome to E37 which is a medical ward for children of all ages. Our aim is to help your child get better and return home as soon as possible. We will try and make the stay for you and your child as pleasant as possible by:

- Welcoming parents to stay with their children.
- Keeping to your child's normal routine with your help.
- Helping you to care for your child as much as you feel able.
- Encouraging normal play and school activities. We have a play leader who is based in the play room. School takes place in term time from 9.15 to 11.45 AM and 1.15 to 3.00 PM.
- Having flexible visiting hours. Brothers, sisters and friends of your child are welcome.
- Allocating one nurse to care for you and your child each shift so that you know who to approach.

Caring for your child

Your child will feel more secure if you carry out the care you would at home, such as bathing and feeding. Your nurse will make sure you have everything you need to do this.

Whenever possible, could you please bring in your own nappies; we will provide a small number of nappies for your child's initial stay. If this is going to be a problem please feel free to discuss this with your nurse.

You may like to help with the nursing care of your child. Please talk to your nurse who will be pleased to support you in this.

Children's mealtimes

Mealtimes are at 8.00 AM, 12 noon and 5.30 PM. When the meals arrive please feel free to collect your child's meal tray. Menus are available in the evening for the following day which you may complete. If your child does not like the food on offer we have a microwave oven for your use if you wish to bring a favourite food of your own.

Telephone

There is a payphone on the ward which will receive incoming and allow outgoing calls. Please ask your relatives and friends to contact you on this number – 421943. It is the responsibility of the parents to answer this telephone. There are more coin box telephones on E Floor by the Children's Intensive Care Unit.

Radio/call button

Behind each bed or cot there is a small box with controls for the bed light, radio and nurse call system. There is also an emergency button to call a nurse urgently.

Doctors

The consultants on E37 are Professor Hull, Dr Rutter and Dr Stephenson. They do their ward rounds at the following times and you are welcome to be with your child when the doctor visits:

9.00 AM Tuesday.
9.00 AM Thursday.
The ward doctors see all the children after 9.00 AM each day.

Facilities for parents

The family care assistants are responsible for looking after parents with the following:

Accommodation
This is available and you may sleep either by your child's bedside or in a room in the Parents' Unit (depending on what is available). You are required to be up and dressed by 8.30 AM. Please keep your room tidy and fold or make your bed each morning.

Meals and refreshments
There is a ward kitchen for staff use and a parents' kitchen opposite ward E38, for making drinks. Please provide your own tea, coffee, milk, etc. For safety reasons we would prefer you not to walk around the ward with hot drinks. There is a non-smoking area at the top of the ward and a smokers' lounge opposite ward E38. Children are not encouraged to go into the parents' sitting room. Parents may use the staff canteen on D Floor. There is also a Women's Royal Voluntary Service canteen on B Floor and a vending machine opposite ward E39. If you are finding it difficult to leave your child to get refreshments, please let your nurse know.

Belongings
You are responsible for your own belongings so please keep your valuables and any medications with you at all times. There are also lockable cabinets in most areas of the ward – ask your nurse for details. Please inform the nurse if you have *any* medications with you for yourself or your child.

Washing facilities

Each side room has a shower and toilet and there is also a shower and toilet on the main ward. There is a washing machine and tumble dryer in the parents' kitchen.

General information

Some children cannot eat, therefore sweets and drinks should be kept inside the locker. Please do not offer other children sweets or drinks unless you have asked their parents' or a nurse's permission.

Portable televisions are available as well as videos that are suitable for all ages.

If you leave the ward please let your nurse know where you are in case the doctors need you or in case the fire alarm sounds.

The shop, hairdressers, post box, citizens advice bureau, bank and cash dispenser, and fruit stall are located on B Floor.

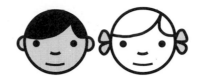

PARENT INFORMATION SHEET

WELCOME TO E40

EMERGENCY ADMISSION

Ward E40 is a children's surgical ward where children have both major and minor operations, planned and emergency. The ward also takes children who have had head injuries or have been involved in road traffic accidents.

On E40 we aim to provide a high standard of care for all our children and their families and encourage a child's family to be involved in all aspects of the child's care. We try to allocate each child with his or her own special or primary nurse, who will help the families plan and carry out each child's care. All the staff however will try to help as far as possible and answer any questions you may have.

Our doctors usually come to see the children each morning and then again late in the afternoon, Monday to Friday. The times do however vary from day to day. On Saturday and Sunday the doctors will come to see the children just once a day.

We aim for all children to be discharged home to their family environment as soon as possible. Children who have had a head injury or bumps and bruises need to stay for at least 24 hours or until they can eat and drink normally and they are back to their normal selves.

Parents are encouraged to stay with their child and we do have facilities to make drinks and snacks, but we do need you to provide your own tea, coffee, bread, etc. Meals can be purchased in the staff canteen or snacks at the WRVS canteen.

If your child is wearing nappies, we ask that you provide these for him/her.

Please do not hesitate to ask the staff for advice or directions whilst your child is in hospital. If we do not know the answer, we will try our best to find out for you.

PARENT INFORMATION SHEET

WELCOME TO WARD E40

PLANNED ADMISSION

E40 is a children's surgical ward admitting children for operations both planned and emergency, major or minor. There are also children in the ward who may have been involved in accidents where they have sustained a head injury.

We aim to give all children and their families a high standard of care planned specifically for each child and to involve the family in all aspects of their child's care. One nurse will plan the care with you.

If your child is being admitted for an operation you are most likely to be asked to come to the ward the day before the operation or on the day of the operation (this depends on a variety of factors and unfortunately not everybody can be admitted on the day of the operation). Children admitted the day before their operation may be able to go home overnight as long as you have no difficulties getting back to the hospital at the time we ask (this may be as early as 7.00 AM). When children are admitted the day before, do *be prepared to stay with us until at least 6.00 PM*. You will have to see two doctors and the anaesthetist and there will be several other children needing to be seen.

On the day of operation we do ask parents/carers to limit visiting to themselves as your child will be recovering from an anaesthetic and will need to rest.

If your child has only a small operation, he/she may be able to go home the same evening. This depends on how he/she is, how you feel and if the doctors agree. Please check with the ward staff when your child is admitted. The doctors will see your child before discharge.

We do provide facilities for you to make drinks on the ward but please bring your own supplies of tea/coffee, etc. Meals can be purchased in the staff canteen if required.

Also, if your child needs any special food/milk, nappies, etc., please bring your own supply into hospital.

PARENT INFORMATION SHEET

WELCOME TO CHILDREN'S INTENSIVE CARE

The Children's Intensive Care Unit is a place where very sick children, or children needing close observation, are cared for. Often just one nurse will look after one child so the child receives the special care he/she needs.

We ask you to ring the doorbell and wait for a nurse before you come in as there may be x-rays being taken or other things happening.

A lot of equipment is used to help your child and this can be very frightening. The staff will always explain what it is used for and this can help to overcome your fear.

If you have any questions at all please ask, as we are always willing to help you. Even though your child is in Intensive Care, he/she still needs you. You can help with some nursing, if you wish, and also read stories and talk to your child. Even though your child may be heavily sedated, it is important to reassure him/her as he/she may still be able to hear and recognize your voice.

The doctors visit the Unit often and we can always arrange for you to talk to them whenever you wish.

There is a kitchen for your use opposite the parents' room and tea, coffee, etc. are provided. There is also a waiting room just outside the door. If you wish for people outside the immediate family to visit, then please talk to the nurse in charge. Too many visitors at once can be distressing, both for children and other relatives, but we will always try to grant your wishes.

Glossary

Activities of Living   Those pursuits and acts related to basic human needs which a person engages in within ordinary everyday life. Some of these are essential for the maintenance of life, whilst others, although not essential, enhance the quality of an individual's life experience, and therefore can be considered to be necessary in order to maintain a complete state of 'health' and well-being.

Associate nurse   The nurse who acts as the primary nurse's deputy when he/she is off-duty, ensuring that care which is planned continues to be delivered in the primary nurse's absence.

Autonomy   The freedom and independence to determine and regulate one's own acts without outside influence or interference. Autonomy is granted when an individual practitioner has attained the required level of knowledge and skills, and has been assessed as competent to practise independently without supervision.

Belief   A firm opinion, feeling or notion which affects how one perceives things to be in reality or how they ought to be ideally. Beliefs underpin the views of individual practitioners about what nursing is and what they are trying to achieve within the caring process.

Caring process/process of caring   The system of nursing and approach that encapsulates the philosophy of nursing care and the means by which a child and family receives the care which has been planned in conjunction with them, and which reflects their specific needs and requirements in relation to the wider influences upon their health and well-being.

Child and family focused care   Recognition that caring for a child also includes caring for his/her whole family, respecting their knowledge about their child and their right to be involved in decision-making and the caring process, thereby enabling them to retain control over their lives.

Community nurse   Someone who aids the child and family's transition from hospital to home, whilst also assisting the family to provide home-based care as an alternative to hospital admission.

Conceptual framework   An idea, view or abstract notion that involves a mental picture or image of a set of related and interrelated objects, properties or events. For example, those concerning the nature of nursing, the role of the nurse, the patient or the environment within which care is delivered.

Holistic   Responding to and treating an individual as a whole person, in a non-fragmented manner, which involves acknowledging the physical, psychological, socio–cultural, environmental and politico–economic context with which they constantly interact, rather than focusing purely upon the symptoms of disease.

Needs   Basic, essential and fundamental requisites or desires that individual human-beings desire or require to live and maintain their 'normal' functioning, i.e. food, shelter, clothing, love and social interaction. The nurse and/or family assists a person to meet these needs if they are unable to do so independently.

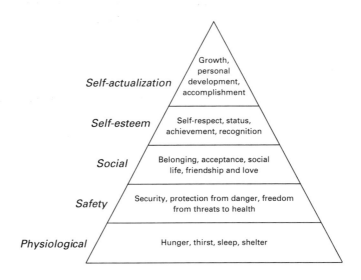

According to Maslow's Hierarchy of Needs [1] (see diagram), higher level needs such as social, self-esteem and self-actualization are only met when lower level ones such as physiological and safety needs have been met. However, individuals have different perceptions of their own needs, which may not necessarily be reflective of the order depicted by Maslow. It is therefore important for the nurse to ascertain not only the child's needs but also the significance of these to the child.

Negotiated care   Refers to a two-way process between the named nurse and child, the parents and family. It is based upon a relationship built upon mutual trust and respect in which each participant is equally valued. The negotiation process leads to a mutually agreed plan of care and level of participation in the delivery of that care which reflects each participant's capabilities and interests.

Process of nursing   A systematic approach to meet the needs of a child and family within the caring process.

Philosophy   A statement related to a set of beliefs and way of thinking with regard to the nature of health and individual human rights, including the principles and values upon which the approach to nursing is based, and the ideologies that reflect the specific needs of children and their families.

Primary/key/named nurse A child and family's 'special nurse' who holds 24-hour responsibility for planning and co-ordinating the delivery of their individual care requirements.

Self-care The means by which an individual person acts on his/her own behalf to prevent illness, promote health, detect disease or provide care/treatment, in order to maintain his/her own 'health' and a state of complete well-being. In the case of paediatrics, self-care may extend to the involvement of a child's parents and family so as to assist in the achievement or maintenance of the child's optimum level of health and well-being.

References

1. Maslow, A. (1954) *Motivation and Personality.* Harper & Row, London.

Index